MAKING THE M(

GILL COX is the Probler
Realm, and is a regular
problems. She also works with the Family Planning
Association. In her work she sees all the time how communication skills and clear, sympathetic information about sex are vital to a healthy relationship.

SHEILA DAINOW is a trained counsellor, who runs groups and teaches counselling skills. She also helps to train Citizens' Advice Bureau workers. The philosophy that underlies all her work is that people must learn to use their personal 'power' to be more in charge of their lives.

This is their second book together. *Making the Most of Yourself* is also published by Sheldon Press.

Overcoming Common Problems Series

The ABC of Eating
Coping with anorexia, bulimia and compulsive eating
JOY MELVILLE

An A–Z of Alternative Medicine
BRENT Q. HAFEN AND KATHRYN J. FRANDSEN

Arthritis
Is your suffering really necessary?
DR WILLIAM FOX

Being the Boss
STEPHEN FITZ-SIMON

Birth Over Thirty
SHEILA KITZINGER

Body Language
How to read others' thoughts by their gestures
ALLAN PEASE

Calm Down
How to cope with frustration and anger
DR PAUL HAUCK

Comfort for Depression
JANET HORWOOD

Common Childhood Illnesses
DR PATRICIA GILBERT

Complete Public Speaker
GILES BRANDRETH

Coping Successfully with Your Child's Asthma
DR PAUL CARSON

Coping Successfuly with Your Hyperactive Child
DR PAUL CARSON

Coping with Depression and Elation
DR PATRICK McKEON

Curing Arthritis Cookbook
MARGARET HILLS

Curing Arthritis – The Drug-free Way
MARGARET HILLS

Curing Illness – The Drug-free Way
MARGARET HILLS

Depression
DR PAUL HAUCK

Divorce and Separation
ANGELA WILLANS

The Epilepsy Handbook
SHELAGH McGOVERN

Everything You Need to Know about Adoption
MAGGIE JONES

Everything You Need to Know about Contact Lenses
DR ROBERT YOUNGSON

Everything You Need to Know about Your Eyes
DR ROBERT YOUNGSON

Everything You Need to Know about the Pill
WENDY COOPER AND TOM SMITH

Everything You Need to Know about Shingles
DR ROBERT YOUNGSON

Family First Aid and Emergency Handbook
DR ANDREW STANWAY

Fears and Phobias
What they are and how to overcome them
DR TONY WHITEHEAD

Feverfew
A traditional herbal remedy for migraine and arthritis
DR STEWART JOHNSON

Fight Your Phobia and Win
DAVID LEWIS

Fit Kit
DAVID LEWIS

Overcoming Common Problems Series

Flying Without Fear
TESSA DUCKWORTH AND DAVID MILLER

Good Publicity Guide
REGINALD PEPLOW

Goodbye Backache
DR DAVID IMRIE WITH COLLEEN DIMSON

How to Bring Up your Child Successfully
DR PAUL HAUCK

How to Control your Drinking
DRS W. MILLER AND R. MUNOZ

How to Cope with Stress
DR PETER TYRER

How to Cope with your Child's Allergies
DR PAUL CARSON

How to Cope with your Nerves
DR TONY LAKE

How to Cope with Tinnitus and Hearing Loss
DR ROBERT YOUNGSON

How to Do What You Want to Do
DR PAUL HAUCK

How to Enjoy Your Old Age
DR B. F. SKINNER AND M. E. VAUGHAN

How to Improve Your Confidence
DR KENNETH HAMBLY

How to Interview and Be Interviewed
MICHELE BROWN AND GYLES BRANDRETH

How to Love a Difficult Man
NANCY GOOD

How to Love and be Loved
DR PAUL HAUCK

How to Say No to Alcohol
KEITH McNEILL

How to Sleep Better
DR PETER TYRER

How to Stand up for Yourself
DR PAUL HAUCK

How to Start a Conversation and Make Friends
DON GABOR

How to Stop Feeling Guilty
DR VERNON COLEMAN

How to Stop Smoking
GEORGE TARGET

How to Stop Taking Tranquillisers
DR PETER TYRER

If Your Child is Diabetic
JOANNE ELLIOTT

Jealousy
DR PAUL HAUCK

Learning to Live with Multiple Sclerosis
DR ROBERT POVEY, ROBIN DOWIE AND GILLIAN PRETT

Living Through Personal Crisis
ANN KAISER STEARNS

Living with Grief
DR TONY LAKE

Living with High Blood Pressure
DR TOM SMITH

Loneliness
DR TONY LAKE

Making Marriage Work
DR PAUL HAUCK

Making the Most of Yourself
GILL COX AND SHEILA DAINOW

Making Relationships Work
CHRISTINE SANDFORD AND WYN BEARDSLEY

Meeting People is Fun
How to overcome shyness
DR PHYLLIS SHAW

One Parent Families
DIANA DAVENPORT

Overcoming Common Problems Series

Overcoming Stress
DR VERNON COLEMAN

Overcoming Tension
DR KENNETH HAMBLY

The Parkinson's Disease Handbook
DR RICHARD GODWIN-AUSTEN

Second Wife, Second Best?
Managing your marriage as a second wife
GLYNNIS WALKER

Self-Help for your Arthritis
EDNA PEMBLE

The Sex Atlas
DR ERWIN HAEBERLE

Six Weeks to a Healthy Back
ALEXANDER MELLEBY

Solving your Personal Problems
PETER HONEY

A Step-Parent's Handbook
KATE RAPHAEL

Stress and your Stomach
DR VERNON COLEMAN

Trying to Have a Baby?
Overcoming infertility and child loss
MAGGIE JONES

What Everyone Should Know about Drugs
KENNETH LEECH

Why Be Afraid?
How to overcome your fears
DR PAUL HAUCK

You and Your Varicose Veins
DR PATRICIA GILBERT

Your Arthritic Hip and You
GEORGE TARGET

Overcoming Common Problems

MAKING THE MOST OF LOVING

Gill Cox and Sheila Dainow

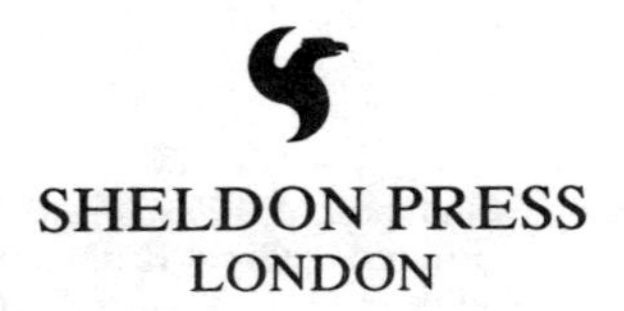

SHELDON PRESS
LONDON

First published in Great Britain in 1988 by
Sheldon Press, SPCK, Marylebone Road, London NW1 4DU

British Library Cataloguing in Publication Data

Cox, Gill
Making the most of loving. —— (Overcoming common problems).
1. Interpersonal relations
I. Title II. Dainow, Sheila III. Series
158′.2 HM132

ISBN 0–85969–566–2

Photoset by Deltatype Ltd, Ellesmere Port, South Wirral
Printed in Great Britain by
Biddles Ltd, Guildford, Surrey

Contents

Acknowledgements

As with our first book, *Making the Most of Yourself*, many have contributed over the years to the thoughts and facts delivered in *Making the Most of Loving*, too many to mention individually. Both of us, though, spent some years working for the Family Planning Association, and their past and present influence and help must be acknowledged, especially Toni Belfield, Medical Information Officer, for her invaluable help and advice.

More personally, we thank Keith, Cyril, Jo and Lee who we love.

This book is also for Laurence, in memoriam.

Introduction

People need people! On a purely practical level, if people didn't come together the human race would become extinct. Clearly, though, people don't only seek to be together for sexual intercourse leading to procreation. We make relationships in order to be reassured of our acceptability, to feel companionship, to feel safer in a world that can seem full of danger. Quite simply, people thrive on being loved.

Psychologists know that humankind needs physical contact for healthy psychological survival. Eric Berne, the creator of Transactional Analysis, called this contact 'strokes', and pointed out that in our particular society people are often deprived of physical contact at a very early age. It's quite unusual for adults in our society to touch each other as part of their ordinary communications – say in business, or on the street, or even in the home. So his idea is that we convert this need for physical contact (which we naturally get as children from mothers, family and other adults), into a need for attention. Each unit of attention equals a stroke, and each of us needs a certain supply of strokes in order to feel happy with our lives.

Making close relationships is the best way of getting strokes. But just because it's a basic human need doesn't make it automatically easy. There are some people who seem to have a life packed with meaningful, and on the whole enjoyable, relationships, and others who find it difficult to start them up, or keep them going.

This book is for anyone who wants to understand more about relationships, or be more in charge of the kind of relationships they have. It's for people just starting out, and for those who have had experience. It's for the young boy or girl, wondering whether they're ever going to meet someone special, as well as those who are older and wonder why they've met many people, but never experienced a satisfying closeness.

We aim to explain why relationships can be difficult, and offer ideas about how to deal with inevitable problems. Some chapters are specifically about sexual relationships, with factual physical information on medical and psychosexual issues, because these are aspects which seem to create enormous anxiety for many people.

However, we hope the book will also be useful and interesting to people who are concerned about other kinds of relationship. Getting on with family, friends, and work colleagues can be just as important, and provide just as many problems, as our more intimate relationships. So the ideas in this book are intended to be of help to anyone who wants to understand and/or improve their way of relating to other people in their lives.

From time to time in the book we've suggested activities or exercises you can do which could help you apply the ideas to your own life. You may want to read the book from cover to cover, or dip into chapters which seem most relevant at the time. You may want to discuss some of the ideas with friends or partners, to help you come to your own conclusions. Use the book in whatever way seems most useful, and enjoyable, to you.

We wish you good reading! Good living! Good loving!

1

So You've Made It This Far

Ask someone what love is and they'll probably have difficulty answering. They may come up with ideas like sharing, caring, having fun, being needed, and being special to someone. They may differentiate love from being 'in love', one being kept for parents, family and friends, the other for their lover. What they'll often forget to mention is that for love to work it requires give and take. It's like a two-way street with an abundance of side-turnings, cul-de-sacs and obstacles — but more about those later.

Essentially, to enjoy love you need to be able to express your care and concern and be open to receiving it. That may sound easy, but if you don't like yourself very much, and so reject anyone who shows an interest in you — on the grounds that any club which wants you as a member can't have very high standards — it will prove difficult. And if you don't even apply for membership in the first place as you don't think you'll ever be considered, it will be still more problematic. On the other hand, it can also be difficult if you've grown up believing you're the most important person in the world and demand respect and care without being willing to treat others with the same thoughtfulness.

In a partnership, each person will have different strengths and weaknesses which may complement each other. However, if you're looking for someone to shore you up because you feel like an incomplete person, or searching for someone to pander to your every whim and gaze at you starry-eyed 24 hours a day, then you're likely to be disappointed in love. Do you know who you are, and what you're looking for?

Who are you? (and how did you get here?)

Have you ever looked in the mirror and wondered who that person really is who's looking back at you? How did you get to be the person you are? Until you have some understanding of that, loving someone else may be a bit like trying to work with your hands tied behind your back. So, who are you? A large part of you will in fact have been determined by other people. You'll have been influenced by many factors, and what happened to you in childhood will have been one of the most crucial. People often wonder why, if they've had bad problems which have warranted seeing a psychiatrist, psychologist or counsellor, so much time is spent discussing the past when their problem is now. The reason is that those formative years can have such a hangover effect.

Starting at the beginning

From the moment we're born we receive messages from our parents, or whoever looks after us. We notice what kind of responses our behaviour gets. We may pick up, for instance, that when we smile our mother smiles back, and that feels good, so we do it again. We may begin to discover that we don't get what we want just because we want it! We start to draw conclusions about what will get us most attention. Is it yelling loudly, being quiet, crying at night, gurgling and blowing raspberries, banging on our cot? As a baby, we need attention to survive, so we learn very fast what will, and what won't, get us that life-giving commodity.

Quite a bit of our learning is done by mimicking what we see around us. Watch a child learning how to speak. It will mimic the words and phrases commonly used at home. If a child decided to make up its own language it wouldn't be understood and would soon be persuaded out of it. So it is with the way we live as well as how we speak. We aren't born with a rule book in our hands which tells us how to get the attention and caring that we need, so we learn the rules of our families very fast. These are the people who have the power to help us survive, so we learn to play the game their way. If we don't, then we can get into a lot of trouble. A baby or child surrounded by huge adults, and for whom even a chair seems like a vast obstacle, seek to learn from the grown-ups.

At baby stage we don't know how to handle anxiety. Babies inevitably experience stress, but have little ability to understand and deal with it. They don't know how to think logically, so they can't sift the evidence and come up with a rational explanation for things which may confuse or worry them. For instance, a baby may sense that Mum is angry, but she may not bother to say, or perhaps it just doesn't understand that she's angry because the washing machine has broken down again, and it's not that the baby has done anything naughty or is being a pain in the neck. If Mum and Dad are often fraught, ill-tempered or inconsistent, a child may blame itself, and hence become anxious about whether or not they're loved at all. Sometimes long-lasting effects can spring from such childhood anxieties.

Who told you that?

At this vulnerable age children are inclined to believe absolutely everything that adults tell them. Eventually they learn there isn't a Father Christmas, but other things stick in the subconscious and become accepted as resident truth. Adults can be wrong, or misinterpreted. A mother, for instance, may have told her son who was exploring his genitals not to touch himself there. She may not have meant *never* touch your penis, but the child may have decided that's what she meant, and feel that the pleasure he experiences is somehow bad and unacceptable. Such a child may experience sexual difficulties as a grown man and even pass on the message to his children. For years women were taught by their mothers that sex was a burden of marriage rather than a pleasure in which they could take equal part. Nice girls didn't, and nice boys didn't ask. Adults' truths can change as society develops different 'norms', but the original message still has a powerful influence.

Along with our parents there will have been brothers, sisters, teachers, and other adults who gave us messages about ourselves, told us what they thought of us, and what they considered to be the 'right way' to behave. We may have chosen some of these messages as examples to follow, or by observing those around us we may assume the same thing will happen to us later. For example:

> Father works hard and is self-sacrificing and his son decides that this is how to be a father.
>
> A little girl is told 'You're just like your auntie', so she decides that she is just like Auntie, so 'I'm thoughtless and selfish, and nobody will like me'.
>
> Mother always puts her family's needs first, she says she's never got time to do what she wants. Her daughter decides that being a mother means it's wrong to want things for herself and finds it impossible to say 'no' to anyone who wants something from her.

If you were repeatedly told things about yourself like 'You're naughty/stupid/rude/silly/too fat/too thin/just like your Uncle Jack and he was always trouble', then you could begin to believe that there was something really wrong with you, and that you would only be acceptable if you changed. Or maybe you were urged to 'Keep at it, and show me when you've got it right', and concluded that you must keep trying to be perfect.

> Joseph started off as an office boy and worked so hard he quickly got promoted, he then impressed the bosses so much with his business acumen that by the time he was 30 he was running a department and in line for a directorship. He worked all hours and his only social life was the occasional drink or meal with colleagues, usually talking shop. To outsiders it seemed the world spread before Joseph's feet. They assumed he could get whatever he wanted and look back on his life and the progress he'd made with great satisfaction and pleasure. However, the message Joseph had received when he was little was that life was a matter of trying hard to find perfection. 'Life is an uphill struggle', his father used to tell him, and of course for Joseph it is. However much he succeeds it will never be enough for him — he'll always need to strive for more.

We've all got thorns stuck in our sides from childhood — and some hurt us more than others.

Not many parents are deliberately malicious towards their children, and most act in the way they think is best for the child. Some may have tried to get their children to live up to their highest expectations and live out their dreams for them, but most will be trying to guide and help rather than trample on their offspring. What parents sometimes forget, though, is that their children believe everything they say, and if they omit the praise and only voice the criticism, or vice versa, then that may be what sticks. Or maybe it's just those bits which are remembered. An actor may get nine good reviews after a performance, but the one critic who writes a scathing review may be the one that lodges in the memory. If you've had some bad reviews from a parent don't let them get out of perspective.

If you were sometimes told you were 'being silly' you may have logged that in the memory. You may not have known exactly what was meant, but if the tone was brisk and critical you would have realized that it wasn't good news. So if you wanted to please your parents, as most children do, you probably tried not to 'be silly', though it's likely this was difficult because you probably weren't told exactly what it was that you *should* do. If you were often put in your place, then you would very soon have got the idea that somehow you weren't quite up to scratch. You might even have developed the notion that you were always going to be a loser because you couldn't do or be whatever it was others thought you ought to. Children who *only* got attention when they were being difficult may have adopted being a 'problem child' as a way of life. It may also have become their role in the family, perhaps taking the heat out of a difficult marital relationship or somehow taking on the family's problems.

> Sharon's parents argued a lot, which upset Sharon. When they weren't arguing her father used to go out, and they'd hardly see him for days. One day Sharon got into trouble for shop-lifting some nail varnish with a friend. They were cautioned by the police and it never went to court, but her father was really angry with her. He was at home though, and he and Sharon's mum didn't seem to be arguing, as they were too concerned about Sharon and what she was doing with her life. Soon Sharon was in trouble a lot. She wasn't conscious of why she was doing it and certainly didn't like forever being in the dog-house at home, and it took the help of a professional counsellor to spot that Sharon had in fact tried to find a solution to her parents' problems and in so doing get some attention from both her parents. Fortunately the problem was nipped in the bud. If the counsellor hadn't spotted the real problem, though, it's possible Sharon would have continued to get into trouble as a way of getting attention for herself and diverting it away from other 'trouble spots'.

All homes will have had their good days and bad days, and most of us will have gained any number of positive traits from our parents. However, because parents aren't perfect, we all approach adulthood with some psychological knocks and bruises which may need attention.

Looking at life from the inside

The psychologist Eric Berne, put forward the idea that each person experiences life from one of four possible viewpoints. He labelled them:

I'm OK — you're OK
I'm OK — you're not OK
I'm not OK — you're OK
I'm not OK — you're not OK

He believed that at a very early age we each decided on whichever of these positions made most sense of our experience of the world, and the messages we received about ourselves.

The idea of being 'OK' means believing you are worthwhile and important to yourself. When you were a baby you might have started off feeling OK, but very quickly you decided that this wasn't the case after all if the all-powerful adults around you told you that you weren't.

Seeing life from the 'I'm OK, you're OK' stance means you will, on the whole, be open, friendly, and feel at home with most people. You generally feel safe, loved and protected. You know in your heart of hearts that you're acceptable, and other people aren't seen as an automatic threat, but all right until proven otherwise. 'I'm OK, you're OK' is like the courteous driver who has confidence in their own abilities behind the wheel, accepts that all drivers occasionally make mistakes (including themselves): they don't have to jostle for position, harass other drivers, or for that matter wait until everyone else has gone, which is what the ingratiator might do. An ingratiator tries to buy love. They feel 'I'm not OK, you're OK'. They've decided that they're not really adequate, worthwhile or important: but everyone else is. Standing in their shoes means constantly feeling small and insignificant compared to others. They will find it difficult to initiate relationships since they can never quite believe that anyone would want to be friends with them or love them.

> Helena has a few friends. Whenever she goes to see one of them she always takes a present and tries to be a good guest while she's there, doing the washing up, helping with anything that needs doing. If a friend ever asks for a favour she never says no, nor will she ever get into an argument with anyone, if someone makes a point she disagrees with she'll always assume that her view is wrong and theirs is right. She never believes that people really want to see her as much as she wants to see them, though she's desperate for someone to love her.

For a different twist there are people who try to overcome feelings of inadequacy by being very competitive, by trying hard to beat other people. They put themselves in the 'I'm OK, you're not OK' position, believe that they're right and everyone else is wrong, bad, or pathetic. In children you can see this come out in the 'My parents earn more than your parents' chat. In adults this could be the competitive driver, the one revving the engine ready to beat everyone else through the lights. They need constantly to prove to themselves that they're better.

> Kevin will never ever admit that he might be wrong, or could have made a mistake. He's pushy and know-it-all and hasn't got time for people who he considers to be weak. However he surrounds himself with friends who are more timid or less bright than he is so that he can always appear superior, at least to himself. His girlfriend is terrified to disagree with him, as when they have had an argument he's not spoken to her for days afterwards, not until she's apologized even if it wasn't her fault.

If life, and their place in it, has seemed really hopeless then a person could decide that no matter what they do they'll never make it, and from the way they look at things everybody else seems to be losing too. If everything seems so pointless then relationships become almost impossible to make because 'what's the point?' This person wouldn't even bother to learn to drive in the first place, believing it was futile, they'd be hopeless, and driving was a dangerous thing to do anyway because the roads were full of lunatics.

> Dan didn't bother looking for a job when he left school because he said he knew he wouldn't get one as 'everyone round here is unemployed' and so no-one would want him. It got so bad he hardly bothered to go out during the day at all and in the evening occasionally went to a local club, but no-one talked to him, and none of the girls seemed to fancy him (and they seemed wet anyway), so that all seemed pointless too, and he stopped going out. Eventually he felt that there was so little in life for him that he might as well die. He felt a victim, unwanted by everyone and everything. Yet Dan had never tried to change things, had never made any efforts on his own behalf as he was in fact paralysed by his own feelings about himself.

In order to develop into adults who are able to accept themselves, and others, we need early messages which establish and confirm that idea. However, if you didn't get them then all is not lost. You can identify the gaps and find ways of filling them for yourself. You don't have to go through life always feeling deprived or inferior.

So, what kind of messages do we need in order to develop an 'I'm

OK, you're OK' perception of the world? The first and foremost is 'Hello and welcome'. From the moment of birth a baby receives information about whether he or she is wanted. If the new arrival is ignored, kept at a distance, or handled with anger, then it's as if the baby is being told it shouldn't exist.

> Sally is an example of how a 'Don't exist' message can stick around. She finds, time and time again, that whenever she makes a friend she begins worrying about how anyone could possibly be attracted to someone like her. She finds it difficult to get close to people because she shuts them out, as her fear makes her go shy. She usually ends up feeling that any failure in a relationship *must* be her fault, whether it is or not.

If you are lovingly touched and cared for when you are a baby it will be easier for you to acquire a sense of self-worth and trust. Parents who have adopted emotionally deprived children often report that cuddles, care and loving can encourage a withdrawn or difficult child to blossom. Such love can make adults bloom too, and some of that you can give yourself, or allow yourself to accept from others you trust.

Can you feel?

Another message it's an advantage to have early in life is 'Your feelings are acceptable'. If your child-like feelings were discounted as unimportant, or inappropriate, then you will find it hard as an adult to express your feelings directly, or even hard to feel anything at all. Inevitably parents pass on some of their own hang-ups, and these are often about expressing anger, love, or touching. Within the family everyone comes to know the rules and rituals, so that, for instance, not expressing feelings seems natural. Things could be very different in the world outside.

> Andrew is a very hard-working serious person. His work colleagues find him reliable and conscientious, but feel uncomfortable with him at any social function. He seems very cut off, very unemotional, and if anyone tries to get close to him he backs off. His parents had always become acutely embarrassed at shows of emotion, whether it was love, frustration or pain — he'd learnt their rules.

Supposing your family found anger difficult to deal with, so it was suppressed? Perhaps you recognize statements like 'You're not angry, you're just tired'; 'Just control yourself, and stop making such a fuss'. If you heard them often enough it's possible you decided being angry is a bad thing. As an adult you may well find that you feel tired at the first sign of anger, rather than accepting you have every right to feel angry with someone or something.

Are you the right sex?

Other people's acceptance of your gender can be crucial. Usually by the age of two or three a child knows what sex it is, and whether this is approved of by the family. In some families, and cultures, boys are seen as a more valuable asset, leaving girls as second class citizens, 'I wanted you to be a boy' can make a girl feel completely rejected, or try hard to be just like the son her father wanted. But boys, too, may discover their sex is a disappointment in the family. Mother may have desperately wanted a daughter with whom to share things, and so may try to make a son fit that role to fulfill her own needs.

How we take to society's sex role stereotyping will also help form the adults we become. Girls may come to feel they should be pretty, slim and dainty. If this doesn't fit at all with their muddied, chubby tomboy behaviour they may rebel, or give in under the pressure.

> Jenny believes she's unattractive. She never really feels at home with other people, and hides herself away in a crowded room. She loathes her body, and dresses to hide as much of it as possible. Her nickname in the family had been 'Ugly duckling'. It was meant to be a joke, but Jenny came to believe it.

Little boys get shoved into particular behaviour, too. They are often told not to cry because it's unmanly, and that showing affection is cissy. It should come as no surprise that a lot of men find it hard to cry, to express frustration or tenderness.

Are you confused?

If you got confused messages you may have been left wondering what on earth you should do. One minute parents might have been saying 'Don't talk to strangers, don't take sweets from strangers, don't let anyone touch you if you don't want them to', and then the next minute insisting you 'Kiss uncle goodbye, be a good girl' even though you may not have wanted to. So, should you say no or shouldn't you? Such quandaries can leave confusion for a long time afterwards.

Those are just some examples of the importance which is attached to those first ideas we gather about ourselves. Our conclusions may be mistaken, or distorted, views of what was or is truly happening. But we get stuck with them, and they are difficult to shake off in later life.

Rewind the message tape

If you don't know already what kind of early messages you received, and whether they are affecting you now, then the following questions may help you find out.

Ask yourself:
What is your earliest memory?
What is the family story about your birth?
Did you have a nickname?
What was your mother's/father's main advice to you?
What did your mother/father say when they were angry with you?
What did your mother/father say to you when they were pleased?
What did your mother/father want you to be?
What do you like most/least about yourself?
Describe the bad feeling you have most often in your life
What would 'heaven on earth' be for you?
If you could change anything about yourself, what would it be?

What was once decided can be re-decided! If you have discovered through reading so far that you made some early decisions which are getting in the way of a fulfilling life for you now, take heart. Things can change.

And there's more

Though the family will have been a prime moulding influence, that's not the end of it. Our cultures, colours, religions, class, all work away, trying to bend us this way or that to get the seal of approval. If a woman's body (or parts of it) are seen as sinful by her religion or her culture, exposing it may cause great shame. Many women in the world are veiled. In some African countries women's clitorises are surgically removed to deny them sexual pleasure. In many cultures, ancient and modern, homosexuality is considered part of the spectrum of sexuality, in other countries it's frowned on. Some religions abhor contraception, others welcome it. Monogamy is the rule in Britain, other cultures allow polygamy. Arranged marriages are the norm for some, for others there's freedom of choice. Divorce is acceptable to some, but not to others. About the only universal cultural taboo is parent/child incest. Just about everything else, from the way we deal with birth and death to the way we eat and love, is different.

So there's the family, culture, religion, colour, class, sex, all pulling this way and that. Add to that the influence of school, your friends, newspapers, magazines, TV and radio, travel, and you'll get some idea of how 'you' were formed. Are you still trying, for instance, to mimic your childhood TV hero?

Check your influences

These questions may help you discover some of the ways in which you may have been influenced by your culture and your early years.

1. *Imagine yourself going back in time. What would life have been like for your ancestors 50 years ago; 100 years ago; 150 years ago?*
2. *Does your culture have strong ideas about work, education, sex, money, death? Can you see ways in which these ideas affect you now?*
3. *When you were a child how did you play? Did you play alone? Did you have playmates? Did you have an imaginary playmate?*
4. *Does the way you play now bear any relation on how you played then? Are your friends and acquaintances similar in any way to your childhood playmates?*
5. *Did you watch TV, listen to radio or read a lot? What were your favourite programmes — comedies, soap operas, serious plays, adventure stories?*
6. *With which characters did you identify? Why?*
7. *Which teacher was your favourite? Why? Is there any way in which that person is still influencing you?*
8. *What was life like at your family tea table? Were you able to contribute equally to the conversation? Was there conversation at all? Did you always get your share? Did everyone seem to ignore you? Is there any way in which you find yourself in the same situations now that you're grown up?*

None of us can totally escape from the influences we grew up with.

Some of them will be so ingrained that it feels like another person sitting on your shoulder saying 'you mustn't do this' or 'you must do that'. Even those voices can become confused. What happens when a cultural 'law' is adjusted, perhaps by immigration to another culture, or religious doctrines reassessed, or social standards shift? Influences can and do change, and you may decide to compromise or negotiate with the voice you grew up with.

What do you choose to believe?

One of the essential elements of being a human being is that we have choice. Having ascertained that many of the things you've been taught are other people's beliefs (and that they can alter) you can then choose which things you wish to believe in.

What were you brought up to believe about the following things?

1. Women should stay at home to look after their children.
2. Girls should stay virgins until they marry, but boys should have sexual experience.
3. There are other types of relationship, like living together, which are as valid as marriage.
4. Contraception and/or abortion are evil.
5. Women are better off without men.
6. Divorce is acceptable if a marriage has irretrievably broken down.
7. The age of consent for female heterosexuals should stay at 16.
8. The age of consent for male homosexuals should stay at 21.
9. If parents divorce children are better off living with their mother.
10. Rape should be a hanging offence.
11. Boys should be the pursuer and ask girls out.
12. Mixed race/religion marriages can't work.

What do *you* believe?

Some of these issues will be determined by law of the land. Of course, you can choose whether to break a law (or rule) or not, taking account of the possible consequences, but much in this list isn't subject to legal stricture, but is a matter of personal values.

To decide what you believe it's advisable to know the facts, to look at both sides of an argument, collect as much information as possible and mull on it for a bit. There is an old saying, 'Those that decide in haste, repent at leisure', and with major decisions in life, or standpoints on moral and social issues you don't have to make snap decisions, so take your time. You may well find that much of what you've been brought up to believe still holds true for you — fine. Indeed, it can be comforting not to have to think about absolutely everything, and choices can be very difficult. There's no need to throw the whole lot away thinking that everything you were brought up to believe is wrong, and that what you should do is completely the opposite of what your parents would have you do, because then you'd be throwing out the baby with the bathwater. You may wish, though, to re-evaluate, moderate some beliefs a little and harden up others.

Remember, too, that as well as changing how you may view social dilemmas, you may also want to change how you think about yourself. Re-evaluating yourself, and the way you relate to others, may make loving friendships a whole lot easier.

Making your own way in the world

Don't get downhearted or defeated if you have identified some things which have put barriers in the way of your being the way you want. You can change. Think back for a moment and remember yourself in the past. You will realize that you have already changed a great deal from the child you may remember. You will inevitably go on changing, and you can influence how.

There are many ways you could go about this. You can do it entirely on your own, or with the help of a partner. You could read up on psychology or use some of the many self-help books available (some of which are listed at the end of this book). You could talk things over with a friend and see if any of their suggestions make sense. There are assertion courses or workshops on various aspects of human behaviour which you could attend (these are often advertised in the press or on local noticeboards). You could choose to work with a therapist or counsellor to help you identify the changes you want to make, and then help and support you through any difficulties. Another option would be to model yourself on someone you admire, learn from their behaviour. This doesn't mean you would become that person, but just as a child learns by watching, so can an adult — if someone else has already cracked the problem, why re-invent the wheel every time?

Stop and think

Before you charge ahead, it's important to remember that wanting to change does not mean you are unacceptable or unlikable as you are. Think for a moment about your friends, or about someone you respect. Can you honestly say they have never made mistakes, that they don't have some irritating habits or are sometimes uncertain about their lives? Knowing this about them doesn't stop you liking or respecting them. This is the kind of relationship you need to have with yourself. Try telling yourself, 'I like myself, and I want to change', not, 'I'll only like myself *when* I change'. If you stick with the latter you'll be approaching the world very negatively, taking the 'I'm not OK' position. The problem with that is however hard you try to hide it, the vibes you put out will be picked up by others. If you don't like yourself, how can you expect others to do so?

When you do feel generally good about yourself (even though you're not perfect), it's likely you'll want to move towards people rather than hide from them. You will want to have friends and make relationships. Not everything will be plain sailing — most relationships have some difficult passages — but other people will no longer have the power to decide how you feel about yourself.

Out in the World After our first relationships with parents, carers and then other close members of the family, we go to school and begin to know people outside our previously small personal world. We have to learn about getting on with others who are equal to us in age and status, and sometimes go through a hard time finding out that we have to share our world with others. We may experience rejection for the first time. It can suddenly become very important to be the same as everyone else in class and agony to be different in any way. Later in life we may be pleased to be, or wish we were, a bit unique and not run of the mill, but it seems we all need to feel we belong before we can branch out independently. There are the joys of finding a 'best friend' or the fear of being singled out by the school bully. All these experiences have some effect on how we continue to make relationships. They all add more material to the script we began creating when we were born.

Growing up can be painful When we hit adolescence we move into a phase of development during which we separate from our parents to become adults in our own right. It's often said these are meant to be the happiest years of your life — piffle! A few sail through without problems, but for most of us it's like climbing the Himalayas and it can seem like an incredible struggle to navigate your way even to the sanctuary of knowing that you will be able to reach the top.

Of course, people have always had to grow up, which is another way of saying growing away from their parents. The word 'teenage' was created in the 1950s in order to identify a commercial market — young people of a particular age group with money to spend. Since then adolescence has been identified as a specific group with specific problems.

Parents find it hard too Growing up can be difficult for both parents and children. Both are having to get used to changes which often happen in fits and starts. One minute teenagers want to be their own boss, the next they want Mum or Dad to take over again and sort out all the problems and tell them what to do. There are likely to be a lot of conflicting needs, both between parents and their teenage children and within the individuals themselves.

> Eleanor has a running battle about what time to come home at night. Her parents want her home by 11.30pm, Eleanor sometimes wants to stay out later and on several occasions has come home late to find her parents waiting for her and they were hopping made. Eleanor feels her mum and dad are being unreasonable as some of her friends are allowed out much later than she is. Her parents say they don't care what other children do, they want to know she's in before they go to bed. There are constant fights about this.
>
> One night Eleanor comes home to find her parents aren't in. She knew they were going out but had expected them to be in and drinking their cocoa when she got there. When they haven't arrived home half an hour after she's arrived she gets really worried and wonders if they've had an accident. When they come in safe and sound and have clearly had a good time at the friends they were visiting Eleanor gets extremely angry with them. Though her parents hadn't intended to teach Eleanor a lesson they inadvertently did so, as she began to understand that their anger might be genuine concern about her. Once she'd acknowledged this they all sat down and discussed yet again Eleanor's 'curfew' and compromised. Eleanor was allowed to come home later at weekends and if she was going to be very late she promised to telephone.

The art of compromise Part of becoming an adult is learning how to negotiate and compromise. This is just one task in the many it seems we have to accomplish before we qualify as adult. Other tasks include becoming economically independent — earning our own living. We have to be able to manage, practically, living separately from our parents. We have to learn how to make and maintain relationships with members of each sex — relationships that may be sexual or non-sexual. We have to develop a set of values, a philosophy. We have to learn how to co-operate with people, some of whom we may not like very much. We have to learn how to plan and set goals and then move towards accomplishing them.

Adolescence is a time of experimenting and discovery. It's a time for 'firsts' — the first date, the first job or move away from home, the first holiday without parents, the first period, the first ejaculation, the first broken heart, the first hangover. It's a time for separating from parents and establishing new connections with peers. One way to look at this is to see it as establishing your own chosen family, and it is true for many people that the friends they form in their teens and twenties become the backbone of their social life.

Few people can manage life completely alone and not many want to be so independent that they are isolated. So when we move away from our parents it is not towards complete independence, but to inter-dependence. This means relating to people on an equal level. As children we're used to life being unequal, with the power in the hands of parents, teachers, big sisters and brothers. The adults have more say than we do, so we learn how to get on by playing the game according to their rules. When we are grown up we have to learn how to share the power, so that there is some give and take. There are those people who never really grow up, the eternal Peter Pans, and it is very difficult for them to maintain adult relationships as a result.

Breaking free The first stage in breaking free of dependence is often rebellion. The rebel, though, is often merely acting against parental or authoritative power. That is not the same thing as self-determination, which is truly deciding what you want and what may be best for you. Rebellion allows you to blame someone else for what is happening to you, because as you are doing the opposite of what someone else wants, they are still effectively making the decisions. Self-determination means taking responsibility for your own actions, and facing the consequences whether pleasant or unpleasant.

Trying new ways of behaving can feel strange. The new way may be better, but still feels peculiar. It's the same when you learn any new skill, be that learning to drive, playing the saxophone or wiring a plug. Getting on with people is also a skill, so it will feel strange if you decide to try behaving differently from usual. Don't let this stop you having a go! Practice will help you establish the change and feel easier and more natural about it.

Other people can lead you only so far — there comes a point when you must find your own direction, make up your own mind. That doesn't mean you have to shut yourself off from other people's help or opinions, isolate yourself in an ivory tower and reject all authority. After all, there are some people it would be foolish to ignore, especially if they have knowledge or skills of benefit to you. For instance, the weather forecaster is likely to be able to predict tomorrow's weather more accurately than you, a car mechanic more likely to repair a noisy engine, a lawyer more likely to know the wisest legal action, and so on. In developing your own ideas about the kind of person you want to be you will inevitably come up against some authority that it is wise to question. For instance, some people gain authority not by virtue of their knowledge or experience as in the examples just given, but through their wish to control others. The 'I'm only doing this for your own good' kind of help, which seems on the surface to be caring, is actually an attempt to control you. Some people believe they are entitled to be more powerful because they are bigger or richer than you — beware of this kind of control! Other people's expertise and counsel can be useful; their control of your affairs is a different matter.

2

The Dating Game

Talking to strangers is dangerous. That's what we're told as children. Of course there are times when caution is necessary and being afraid is reasonable. But there are times when we *do* want to talk to a stranger, to chat up someone to be our friend or perhaps something more special, so why should fear strike then? Fear and anxiety are sensations we're all familiar with. The stomach 'drops', the body tenses, starts to sweat and shake, the pulse races with the mind. You know the feeling!

The basic mechanism of why this happens takes us way back into human history. When the human organism was evolving back in prehistoric times, it had to develop a way of surviving any threat to its life. Remember that at that point in human development things were very simple. If there was some threat to survival the human organism could do only do two things — either stay to fight or run away. So the body created a very efficient way of mobilizing its resources in order to fight or run. Hormones, predominantly adrenalin, are released into the system, and they raise the level of tension in the muscles and make the heart beat faster. Blood is pumped quickly to the limbs and head — the head is needed in order to analyse the threat, the arms and legs in order to fight or run. The breathing gets faster to pump oxygen to all the body. All this bodily activity creates heat, and the body's cooling system comes into operation producing sweat.

Now, this is a very efficient system for the comparatively simple situation of either confronting or running away from a life-threatening problem. Faced with a rampaging dinosaur, or a racing car heading straight for you, your body would probably swing you into action. The problem is that we live in a very complicated society. Most of the threats we experience aren't ones that we can easily run away from or meet head on because it's not only our lives at stake. We can be afraid of losing love, companionship, self-esteem or status, as well as more material things like money, housing, food and so on. Whenever we perceive we're in danger of losing something that's valuable to us, though, the body still goes into stress response — we get ready to fight or run. Such responses may be recognized as fear, anxiety, anger, excitement or sorrow.

The physical response to a threat is often accompanied by familiar thought patterns. It can be as if the mind has a screen, and on it we project great disasters. For instance, you may see yourself suggest a date to someone and then see them reject you in an offhand way. If you are very good at making up such scenes in your head you will go on to see the whole world rejecting you and leaving you alone and friendless. The fear will get worse. A familiar internal voice may remind you that 'you'll never succeed', 'don't get too close, or they'll find out just how awful you really are', 'why should anyone like you, you're too short/ugly/old/young/fat?'

Social rules can create fears. Social acceptability can be very important to people, they like to 'fit in' somewhere — with family, friends, religious group, political group or whoever. Groups tend to make their own membership rules and if being drummed out of the Brownies would be really upsetting and a great loss then you may think twice about breaking those rules or codes of conduct. But it's not only groups you've chosen to belong to that may be making up your rule book. Some may have been handed down to you from the past. For instance, in the nineteenth century, social rules meant that 'nice girls' waited to be asked to 'step out'. Few women would have wished to be thought of as 'forward'. Sometimes these hangovers from the past get caught in our rule book, and affect how we see the world now.

Try this exercise:
Work out which year your parents would have been in their late teens, and think about the social rules which would have governed their lives — how they would meet, and so on. Then note down anything you think they may have passed on to you, directly or indirectly. Then think about when your grandparents were teenagers, and what they may have passed on to your parents.

Shifts in social attitudes affect the rules too. In very recent history there have been major changes in social expectations. The Women's Rights movement, for example, has been responsible for a different perception of women's role in modern society. In a multi-cultural society like Britain new influences come into play. The growth of the media, television and radio, means that we have considerably more information about different lifestyles than our grandparents would have done. Even things we take for granted, like women's magazines, have only been widely available in the last

80 or so years. Increase in travel can widen experience. All of these things have an effect on our expectations, and the options we have available to us. Trying anything new can be frightening, though, be it a new idea, a new style of clothes, the first foreign trip, starting a job or hang-gliding. All can make you feel sick with excitement or panic.

Asking someone for a first date is taking a risk. You can feel very vulnerable because you are opening yourself up a little, and rejection can be painful. Someone may just not fancy you very much, or may be so shy themselves that they do nothing to help you along, or have other personal reasons why they turn you down. It's important not to over-dramatize such rejections. They are not a threat to your very survival, nor are they part of a master plan to ensure that you are left alone in the world!

The skill used when approaching someone will affect your chances of success. Making friends and having fulfilling relationships with people has quite a lot to do with skill, and skills are learnt, they aren't inborn.

Breaking the ice

The first few minutes can be the most difficult, especially if you find that you get tongue-tied through anxiety. Here are some guidelines which may help you over the fear barrier.

Listen to yourself

Imagine this scene. You're at a party. You see someone very attractive and make your way over to them. You introduce yourself and begin a conversation. After a minute or two, the person looks over your shoulder, smiles at someone else, and brushes past you. What are you thinking and feeling as a result of this event?

Are you calling yourself names such as 'boring', 'ugly', 'fool'? Are you finding fault with yourself — 'I should have guessed they wouldn't want to talk to me', 'I was too forward', 'I should have waited for someone to approach me'? Did you expect them to leave, are you thinking 'I knew it would turn out like this', or 'This kind of thing always happens to me'?

Analyse the messages you're giving yourself. Those names you call yourself are like labels you put on yourself. Then you judge yourself according to the label, without even listening to the evidence. What's more, you find yourself guilty!

Try this exercise:
Make a list of all the labels you give yourself. Then write down by the side of each one a description of what actually happens.
For example: I'm shy = I get anxious when I meet new people
I'm no good at talking to people = sometimes I can't think of things to say
I'm too short = I'm 5'2" tall
I've got no friends = I don't have as many friends as I'd like
I'm too fat = I'm 12 stone
When you do it this way, you give yourself evidence rather than a judgement.

If the evidence tells you there are things about yourself you want to change, then you can set about doing it. Telling yourself, for instance, that you're ugly will only depress you, since once the judgement is made there isn't a lot you can do about it. However, if you tell yourself 'I've got brown eyes, a nose, a mouth, straggly hair, crooked front teeth,' etc, then you can begin to distinguish the things you can change from the things you can't, or wouldn't wish to because you're happy with them. You will have to learn to live with those things that cannot be changed, but you can work on the others. You could, for instance, get a good haircut to make the best of your hair, get your teeth fixed, and vow to remember that you've got interesting eyes.

One thing about these changes, though, is to make sure you're doing it for yourself, not because you think you ought in order to please other people. You can't guess what will please other people. Features of yourself you loathe they may love, or vice versa. Also be careful that you're not hiding from emotional conflicts by scapegoating a part of your anatomy. Blaming your crooked nose for the fact that you don't have any friends is a way of not taking your share of the responsibility for what happens between you and others. Relationships won't change dramatically if all you do is get your nose cosmetically altered, without also changing your willingness to take that responsibility.

Jumping to conclusions about what other people may think of you by judging yourself negatively is a habit that can be hard to break.

Here is another exercise which may help:
Make a list of all the things you're proud of having achieved in

your life. Start with being born — that was your first achievement! You learnt to eat, to walk and talk — more tremendous accomplishments. Include anything you can think of, nothing is too big or too small. Other examples might be learning to drive, or to swim, making a friend, cooking a meal. Don't stop yourself by listening to your inner critic telling you that boasting is bad. Let yourself go!

Of course your critic is right in a way, because if you were to repeat this list to everyone you met they would soon get bored with you. Bragging is not the same as self-assurance. But it can be just as bad never to admit, even to yourself, that you've achieved a great deal and so can, if you wish, achieve some more.

If you feel you need a reminder that you're not so bad after all, then you could write a list of some of your achievements so that you can refer to it when you're being hard on yourself.

Watch yourself

One of the easiest ways of turning people off is by body language. Whatever we're actually saying with our voices and words, our bodies are also giving out a message. When these two messages conflict, trouble begins. For instance, someone who has labelled themselves as 'ugly' will shrink away from people, avoid eye contact and keep their head down. The message that comes across from the body language is 'I'm not worth bothering about' even though the words might say 'Would you like a dance?' If you tell people, by whatever means, that you're not worth a second look then why shouldn't they believe you? So become aware of your body — look at yourself in the mirror, look at photographs of yourself. Make yourself conscious of how you're standing, what you're doing with your arms and hands. If your body is used to its old language, you may have to teach it a new one.

Again, you may have a little voice inside you saying, 'But that's vain'. Just as bragging is not the same as self-assurance, so self-awareness is not the same as conceit.

Watch other people

Another way of becoming aware of the importance of body language is to notice the effect other people have on you, and each other. Watch people who are comfortable in social situations, and compare them with others who aren't. When you're watching films or plays notice how actors can communicate with their bodies. Have some fun pretending you're an actor in various roles and see how you'd move.

Move in Standing on the sidelines and being a wallflower won't get you anywhere except pasted in when they come to redecorate. If there are individuals or groups you want to talk to then move towards them, rather than waiting for them to come to you.

Lean Leaning towards people you're with shows interest. Leaning back with your arms crossed across your chest may tell them that you're bored or feeling critical.

Look Eye contact is important. If you don't look at someone at all while you're speaking to them then you will come over as shifty. If you stare at them without dropping your eyes occasionally then they'll feel uncomfortable. If you're very nervous of looking people in the eye, try focusing on a spot in the middle of their forehead — they'll think you're looking at them.

Smile If you smile at someone they feel welcome, it's that simple. Think how you feel when someone spontaneously smiles at you (providing you're not assuming they must be laughing at you!). Smiling lights up the face and encourages people to believe that you want to make contact with them. If you go overboard and become like the proverbial Cheshire Cat then you'll diminish your own impact though, so again the aim is for balance. If you smile constantly, even when you don't mean it, then the message you may end up giving is 'You don't have to take me seriously' or 'I'll smile through anything'. Neither should be true.

Respond Let your face and body show your responses — nod, frown, smile and so on if you're enjoying talking to somebody. If you look wooden and unresponsive the other person is likely to think you're not interested, and that they're boring you.

Touch A brief touch on the arm or shoulder often conveys a great deal of warmth and liking. Not so brief that you give the impression you've just burnt your fingers, not so long that the other person thinks you're moving in on them too much, and not so often that people get the impression you're putting on a show. To help you get it right practise in front of a mirror, even better is to get someone to tape you with a video camera and play that back to yourself.

So, you're through the first few minutes. What next?

Begin at the beginning

We've already looked at the excuses you could find for yourself not to bother talking to someone you're interested in. But now you *are* going to bother. When it comes to the crunch there is only one way to start a conversation, and that's by talking. There are some tried and tested ice breakers — 'Hello, what's your name?', 'Do you live near here?', 'Would you like a drink?'., 'Did you enjoy the film?', 'How are you?'. These are an easy way to start off. Their disadvantage is that because they are ritual questions the other person can give quite a short answer, and leave you having to think of something else to say.

Another way of starting off is to talk about something you've noticed, either in your surroundings or in yourself. So, when you're not sure how you'll approach someone, take a moment to look around and ask yourself:

'What's happening now?'
'What do I notice about the other person?'
'What am I thinking and feeling?'
'What do I notice around me?'

This will help you focus on something you can talk about.

> Simon, finding himself next to a very attractive woman at a party, focused his mind on how difficult it was to concentrate on holding his plate and his glass of wine, and dodge the people trying to get past them. Many things here could give him a beginning. 'Hello, I've just decided the only way to manage is to grow a third arm. You look well-organized — how do you do it?' or 'This makes me feel as if I'm on the Underground' or 'Careful that in the balancing act you don't spill wine down your terrific outfit'.

There are lots of ways you can start off a conversation. Here are a few more suggestions:

Asking for information 'Is there somewhere around here that has good food?'

'Can you recommend a good doctor? I've just moved in and need to register with a practice.'
'This is my first time here, do you know how to get to . . .'

Giving compliments 'I love the way you've matched those colours — they look wonderful.'
'You've done a really good job on that, you deserve to be proud of yourself.'
'I see you've got good taste in books/records (or whatever).'

A word here, too, on accepting compliments. If someone pays you a compliment try not to be dismissive with 'Oh, this old thing' or 'Any idiot could do it' or you may inadvertently make the complimenter feel small for trying to be nice to you.

Making a joke 'By the time you get served here they may as well read you the last rites as well.'
'Have you heard the joke about . . . ?'

Discussing the news 'Have you heard the latest about . . . ?'
'What do you think about . . . ?'

Commenting on the surroundings 'I love this music, don't you?'
'Do you find it a bit stuffy in here?'
'Look at that . . .'
'Can you smell . . . ?'

Talking about something you've done recently and enjoyed 'I was very impressed by a play I saw last week.'
'I've just come back from . . . I had a wonderful time doing/seeing . . .'
'I watched . . . on the TV last night and . . .'

The direct approach Another possibility is to share your thoughts and feelings with the other person by saying something like:

> 'I'd like to talk with you for a while; I find you very interesting and would like to get to know you a little better.'

This is a bit more risky of course. You're more open to rejection than with the ritual conversation openers suggested above, but it could turn out to be more rewarding. After all, you will both know that you're interested in more than a few minutes of polite chit-chat.

Taking it further

Once you've started, the next task is to develop a good conversation. If you listen to two people enjoying a really good chat you'll notice that each one does some listening and some talking. What's happening is that they are listening to each other in an active way, and prompting each other to continue, often by asking questions and sharing information about themselves.

When you listen actively, you concentrate more on the other person than on yourself, and check out with them that you understand them. Checking is often done by repeating in your own words what the other person has said. In this way you reflect to the other person that you do, or are trying, to understand them. They'll feel reassured and encouraged to go on talking.

This kind of listening means that you give the other person a great deal of attention, not just wait for them to finish so that you can say your twopenneth, air your views, or judge what they say as right or wrong, good or bad.

You have ways of making them talk

Questions which encourage people to go on talking are called open questions. They cannot be answered with one or two words. Those kind of questions are called closed questions.

If you ask someone 'Where do you live?' they could answer 'Leeds'. If you follow that up with 'Do you like Leeds?' the answer could be 'Yes' or 'No'. To continue the conversation yet another question or observation will have to be aired, making it all quite hard work. However, if you were to ask 'What are the good things about living in Leeds?' it will be harder to just give a one word answer, they're more likely to give you some information, such as 'I'd prefer to live in York but my family are in Leeds', or 'Yes, because I live near a big park and that's ideal for the dogs and the people around are nice'. Now, you could go on to talk about York, family, dogs, walking — you've been given several bits of free information to pick up on. The response to an open question usually includes some free information. Listen out for this, because these are clues about things you can go on to talk about.

Open questions usually begin with phrases like:

'How do you feel about . . . ?'
'What do you think about . . . ?'

'What do you like/dislike about . . . ?'

The more you listen and prompt in this way, the more the other person will believe you're interested in them. Apart from anything else most people are enormously flattered by that amount of attention — wouldn't you be?

And how about you?

If you don't want a conversation to become a one-sided interrogation, then you will have to give something, too. It's the willingness to reveal information about yourself that moves a casual chat towards intimacy. If you're unable to share information about yourself, your contacts will never get past the superficial.

If you find it difficult to talk about yourself, and many of us do, then here is an exercise which may help:

List all the important things which have happened to you so far in your life. These might include childhood events, school, career, travel, your first job, your first girl/boyfriend, people who have had some significant influence on you, losses you've experienced, hobbies, books you remember reading, films which have left an impact on you, times when you've been especially angry, frightened, happy or sad, and so on.

This will provide you with ideas for things you can share in a conversation.

Sharing things about yourself doesn't mean you have to reveal all your innermost secrets. At the beginning of a relationship you will probably only want to disclose neutral information about yourself — your job, holidays and so on.

When you want to deepen the contact you could begin to talk more about personal thoughts and feelings. This exercise might help with this:

Complete these sentences, either in writing or preferably by speaking into a tape recorder:

Something I believe in strongly is ....
I feel sad when I think about ....
If I could have three wishes I'd ....
What most frightens me is ....
I've always wanted to ....

What I'd most like to happen in future is ....
One of the best times in my life was ....
What makes me most angry is ....

Add more sentences if you want to.

If you're not used to talking about yourself, this kind of practice will help make it easier for you. Don't worry about feeling self-conscious. Each time you speak into your tape recorder, or repeat aloud what you've written, it will become easier, and soon it will feel quite natural.

As with so many of the things we're suggesting, you may have to over-ride that voice in your head which tells you 'Boasting is bad', 'No-one would be interested anyway', 'The other person is more important.'

We're not suggesting that each time you meet someone, you launch into a well-rehearsed monologue of your entire life history and opinions about everything. That will be just as likely to invite a brush-off as saying nothing at all. Our proposals are based on the knowledge that good conversation, and eventually a good relationship, depend on each person being willing to take responsibility for keeping their part of it. You should take neither more nor less. If you take more, then the other person will in time feel overwhelmed and controlled. If you take less, the other person might eventually get resentful at having to do all the talking.

If you wanted to make the contact between you more intimate, you could share your feelings about what's happening between you. This means saying what attracts you about the person, what may irritate you about them, how you feel about them now, telling them what fears or hopes you have, and talking about what you want.

Shall we meet again?

So far we have pretty much concentrated on the first stage of contact. Let's suppose that you've successfully negotiated this first step, have enjoyed talking with the person, and know that you would like to see them again. What now?

The most sensible and logical thing to do would be to tell the person how much you've enjoyed meeting them, and that you would like to meet again. You could suggest a specific meeting for a meal, a night at the cinema, the theatre, a party, somewhere which would be enjoyable for both of you.

Realistically, though, it may sound simple, but for some people this is exceedingly difficult. That same voice with those same old messages gets in the way. 'They won't want to spend time with me', 'They're only speaking to me out of politeness', 'It's too forward'. Instead of asking for yourself, you may wait for the other person to make a date.

Who should do the asking? One problem women have in our society is an old-fashioned but still quite strong social code which says that men should do the asking, while women should do the waiting. If a girl would like to ask a boy for a first date, she may fear running the risk of being seen as 'aggressive', 'pushy', in some way 'unnatural'. What may not be so obvious is that this is actually also a problem for many men. Just because they are 'supposed' to take the lead doesn't mean they are necessarily happy about it, or able to do it.

These unwritten social rules, even though they're a hangover from the past, still influence us. If you don't believe in them, then don't let them stand in your way too much. After all, if a girl wants to get to know a particular boy better, and he doesn't take the initiative himself, she won't be any worse off than she is now if she approaches him and it doesn't work! Her hopes may be dashed, but she's also then free to leave that dream and try the next one.

Take heart from this letter written to a magazine Problem Page:

> I thought I'd write to you, because I've actually had my problem solved! I met a girl I really fancied and wanted to ask her out. We ran into each other quite a lot, but she always seemed to have friends around her, and I thought she wouldn't be very interested in me. I resolved on lots of occasions to ask her out, but when the time came I was always too nervous, and we only exchanged smiles. Last month she asked me! Since then we've seen a lot of each other and it's great. I wanted to write this letter because I think there are a lot of young men like me who are really fed up with always having to take the lead and perhaps this will encourage other girls to ask a bloke out.

The brush off

So far in this chapter we've dealt with developing an encounter which assumes that your approach is successful. It won't always be.

There is always a risk of a brush-off, so it's as well to be prepared in case.

Don't expect too much If you approach each new contact as if it's the ultimate test of your acceptability or lovability, you are setting yourself up for potential disappointments. There will be some people who don't like you — no-one gets on with everybody. Sometimes people you approach simply don't have the energy or space in their lives to cope with a new person at that particular time.

Don't expect too little (of yourself) You may be giving yourself 'turn-off' messages like 'How could anyone see anything in me', 'I'm not attractive enough', 'They'll think I'm pushy'. All these thoughts put you in the 'I'm not OK' position. Try, instead, to look upon situations like this as opportunities to learn something about yourself. If you're very anxious try to think of yourself as an observer and be curious rather than frightened of what will happen.

Don't assume the worst Imagine someone you don't know very well has asked you for a date. Make a list of as many reasons as you can think of for possibly wanting to turn them down. Examples might be a prior engagement, not feeling very well, having to work, being involved in some emotional upset. If you look at the list you've made you'll see that very few of the reasons are likely to relate to the other person's intrinsic worth, after all how could they? You don't know the person well enough to do that.

There are many reasons why you might be turned down. If you always assume that any rejection is a rejection of you, then you're bound to get distressed. That kind of 'mind-reading' will cause you trouble, since you'll assume the worst interpretation of events. The probability is that if someone doesn't want to take up a date with you, the reasons will be as much or more to do with them as with you. Their lifestyle, present situation or mood may mean they're just not open to starting a new relationship. That's not your fault.

If they've said no

If you get a brush-off, what do you do? First, be curious about your reaction. Don't just feel it, but observe it. Make yourself aware of how your body is reacting and what you're thinking. This will help you stop the negative voice which starts up in your head telling you just how terrible you are, and how you should never have bothered trying in the first place as it was a complete waste of time.

Make sure you've heard right. *Listen* to what the other person has actually said, and reflect back to them what you hear, so you don't jump to wrong conclusions. For instance, if you ask someone to meet you tomorrow night, you may be so relieved at actually having asked them that you'll only hear them say 'No, I don't want to go out with you' when they've actually said 'No, I can't manage tomorrow evening'.

Share your response to what they say — not in order to change their mind (although it may do that!), but as a way of reminding yourself that they are not responsible for your reaction to their reply. If you're disappointed then say so. Whether you decide to take it on the chin or sink into deep depression is your choice. Once you accept this it will help you feel less controlled by other people. You could say 'I'm disappointed you won't go out with me. I feel a bit foolish for having asked but I'll survive.'

Ask about anything you don't understand. If you genuinely don't understand the reasons for the rejection it's better for you to know than to spend hopeless hours trying to work it out, probably imagining the worst. So you could ask if they would be willing to tell you why they've said no. The other person may choose not to tell you — and that's fair enough. However, if they do, you may learn something about yourself that you could begin to change if you chose. If someone says they don't find you attractive, take care not to overdramatize that to yourself. They aren't saying you're the ugliest person in the world, no-one could possibly fancy you — or whatever your internal story-teller scripts for you. The situation is that he or she, one person, doesn't fancy you. It's disappointing, but it isn't a tragedy, so don't make it one.

Negotiate for further contact, if you want to. The other person may not want a deep relationship with you, but may be interested in something less intense. 'I understand that you don't want to see me as often as I would like, but could I phone you every now and again for a chat?'

Accept that the other person, just like you, has an absolute right to make relationships with whoever they choose. They also have a right to refuse any explanations if they don't want to give them. Sometimes you need to be graceful about taking no for an answer. It's a waste of energy to keep banging your head against a brick wall.

Accept your feelings

Inevitably a brush-off leaves a touch of sadness. After all, you've lost something. Even if the relationship never got off the ground, you've lost the fantasy you had about it. Let yourself feel that sadness, and then move on. If you find that you're sunk in a deep depression, or overcome by intense anger or fear for a long time, you need to ask yourself who you're really grieving for? Sometimes feelings that we have never expressed, maybe disappointment, fear or anger from way back in our personal history, get triggered off by current events. It's as if by repeating them we can somehow resolve them. And so a simple refusal for a date can turn into a major tragedy.

Back to the asking

Remember that the manner in which you ask will make a world of difference. Expect to be rejected and you probably will be, because you'll go about it in a ham-fisted way. On the other hand, an arrogant approach may solicit a forceful rebuff.

When you want to say no

To be in control of your own life means you need to be able to say no to things you don't want to do. If you feel you have to say yes to everyone who has plucked up the courage to ask you, even if you don't fancy them or like them very much, or have umpteen other things to do, then you throw away your own control. Wanting to be liked by everyone can lead into impossible situations, and sometimes it's just not possible to avoid upsetting people, just as you may have been unavoidably upset.

We human beings are sometimes frightened of controlling our own lives and accepting responsibility for them. Facing what needs doing can sometimes be incredibly difficult, and even painful, but if you can face things then there's a chance of sorting them out. If you hide painful facts from yourself the need for control may show in other ways. The eating disorders — anorexia, compulsive eating and bulimia nervosa (bingeing and vomiting) — are often triggered by a need for control. The anorexic wastes away forcefully refusing things, but refusing what's good as well as bad. The compulsive eater tends to hide behind a wall of fat. It presents a chance for them to blame something else, an excuse for not doing much about their own problems, and yet feel guilty about any nourishment they take. The bulimic also exerts iron control, but never quite where they want to. Phobias, obsessions, psychosomatic illnesses, migraine —

there are many emotional and physical conditions that can be brought on by stress. And stress can be caused by feeling unable to say either yes or no when you want to. You have every right to your own behaviour, providing you also accept responsibility for it.

If you do want to say no to someone who is making friendly overtures, then do remember that they've got feelings too. They're not more important than yours, but there's no need to be spiteful and crush their ego. Appreciate it's taken guts to ask, and it is a compliment. If you have reasons you'd like to explain for not taking up the person's offer then tell them, as it may stop them over-dramatizing your rejection of them. For instance, you could say 'I really appreciate you asking me. It isn't possible for me to accept because I don't have the time at the moment to make a new friendship.' Or '. . . thank you for asking. I don't think we have enough in common to make time together really enjoyable.'

Love hurts

Making and breaking relationships can be a painful business. Although you may get hurt sometimes, if you never take risks you also never experience the heights, the pleasures and rewards that good friendships and good lovers bring. Though it doesn't feel like it at the time, painful experiences aren't always totally bad. Sometimes you can find, after you've been through the pain, that you understand yourself or others rather better, and that this in itself is helpful. Bear that in mind.

Love at first sight

Hundreds of songs have been written about this phenomenon — and it certainly sounds terrific. Suddenly you see someone across a crowded room, and time stands still, your eyes meet and you know this is the person for you. Of course, it's possible to feel intensely attracted to someone the first time you see them. Even though it seems like a magic moment, you are in fact bringing to it a great many expectations and assumptions triggered by the appearance, behaviour, posture and voice of the other person. You bring your history to the encounter, just as the other person brings theirs.

A fascinating exercise is described by psychologist Robin Skinner, in his book *Families and How to Survive Them* which he wrote with John Cleese. A group of people who have never previously met are asked to join up with people in the room who either remind them of someone in their family, or make them feel they would have filled a gap in their family. They do this without speaking to each other, going purely on intuition. Surprisingly enough, it turns out that people always gravitate to those whose families functioned in very similar ways to their own. For instance, they may be similar in that their families found difficulty in sharing affection, expressing anger, or perhaps a parent was absent. We seem to have ways of identifying types of people, and are often attracted to others through some sub-conscious reckoning. However, being attracted to and loving are quite different. One may lead to the other, but love takes work.

True love's dreams

Many people at some point in their lives decide that they would like to live with a partner, and finding the right person can prove a difficult task. In Western society the popular view of these intimate relationships follows the myth of romantic love. Anyone who has watched television or film romance, or read a Mills and Boon romantic novel, will recognize this powerful myth.

The first rule of romantic love, as myth has it, is that it is immediately recognizable. 'When you meet the right person you'll know', 'I was swept off my feet'. The second rule is that this romantic love is powerful — 'Love will overcome all obstacles'. The strongest rule is that it is everlasting — 'And they lived happily ever after'. Fairy stories told us in childhood, and all the rules they seem to impart, can have a lingering effect.

Mingled with these rules are the things we picked up about relationships from the example of our parents, authority figures, older brothers and sisters. All children have a natural urge to experiment and explore their world, though some of these urges are discouraged. Maybe we were told who we could or could not play with: 'Don't play with those rude dirty children'. We may have been punished for getting dirty, or only praised when we were clean: 'Don't play in that mud', 'You're so dirty, go and wash those disgusting hands', 'You do look pretty — come and give mummy a kiss'. Most little children have a great fascination with their own bodies, and some learn that there are certain things their parents don't want them to do or talk about. Common unmentionables include faeces, masturbation, genitals, and urination.

In addition to physical unmentionables, many of us will have learnt that some feelings were more acceptable than others. 'Don't sit there with a long face', 'If you're going to shout like that then you can go to your room', 'It's very silly to be afraid'. People don't say these things in order to give you problems later, they say them because they think they'll be helpful. However, each statement is a denial of the real feeling the child is experiencing. If a child learns that mummy or daddy doesn't like anger or sadness they may well decide to hide their feelings, and pretend to be happy, and many of us do just that in relationships we feel are important to us.

As if this weren't enough to contend with, the myths of romantic love can compound the difficulties of facing what loving someone truly involves. Does any of these ring a bell with you?

Some day my prince will come
Falling in love is wonderful
There must be someone for me
Love is the only thing
Love is forever
If you really loved me, you'd know what I wanted
True love
As long as we've got each other everything will be fine
Without love you're nothing

These myths are really about 'being in love', not about love itself. They promote the idea that to be alone is frightening, shameful and a sign of failure, and that the solution is to search for a partner and then all will be well. Even though the false nature of this idea is evident in the increasing divorce rate and the introduction of easier divorce laws, its powerful influence remains. People continue to search for the ideal partner and believe romantic love to be the peak of experience.

The expression 'being in love' have existed since human beings developed the ability to describe emotions. The Song of Solomon in the Bible, or some of the great love stories which are part of Greek and Roman mythology stand as proof. But the development of these ideas into a set of values and rules for a love-life only date back in Western culture to the 13th century. One popular theory is that Eleanor of Aquitaine, tired of the rude and boorish behaviour of her knights and soldiers when they were at her court rather than fighting a war, drew up a manual of rules about how men were to behave towards the female sex. *The Art of Courtly Love* set out a code of conduct emphasizing the importance of gallantry and courtesy. Women were to be seen as idealized figures symbolizing purity and modesty. Relationships between men and women were supposed to aim for an 'eternal oneness, undying devotion', and would inevitably be full of agony and ecstasy.

This seems a bit high-flown nowadays, but it's possible to see how strongly these ideas still influence our ideas about loving relationships. Films like *Gone with the Wind* and *Casablanca* were made decades ago, but still fill the cinemas when they return, which they do with monotonous regularity. People flock to see them not so much for their superb cinematography but for their 'romance'. Their stories basically are about unrequited love with the 'perfect' partner. We never know whether Scarlett manages finally to get together with Rhett Butler, although the inference at the end of the film is that she's going to do her level best. Audiences for *Casablanca* have shed many a tear at the thought of Humphrey Bogart watching the plane carry away his true love! Despite all the efforts of the feminist movement, these stories are still attractive to many people.

Modern romantic fiction is big industry. Most women's magazines have their share, and there are even entire magazines devoted to escapist romance. Each year 25 million books are sold by Mills and Boon alone, most of which are pure romance. They follow a predictable formula, along the following lines. Young woman meets young man, preferably somewhere exotic. The man is likely to be the broody, mysterious type and he ignores her/treats her like a sister/misunderstands her. She gets into danger or difficulty, he rescues her and realizes he loved her all the time! Nowadays such fiction doesn't end with the words 'and they lived happily after' but the idea is the same.

The myth of romance is that it offers certainty, excitement, and a solution to all problems once you have found the 'right' person. If you approach your relationships believing the myth to be true you're in for a big disappointment. Romantic love can be wonderful and exciting, but it can also cause sadness, and anger. The idea that if you love someone, and they love you, so all will be perfect is a trap. If you fall into it every disagreement will leave you miserable and you will be unable to recognize the truth that relationships do not magically become successful and fulfilling — they develop through a commitment to jointly solving problems and sharing both good and bad times.

Anyone who has been in a loving relationship for any length of time will tell you that the romantic fiction view of love has little to do with the real world. The passion of sexual attraction can make it seem as if a particular person is the ideal partner, and under this illusion many couples marry or live together. When the passion begins to fade the ideal partner turns out to be just another human being after all, with faults and insecurities and difficult habits to live with.

To ensure a lasting relationship the people in it need to be able to cope with change, and we'll deal with this in the next chapter. Relationships with the best chance of success view conflict and change as opportunities for growth rather than reasons to avoid getting involved at all. People in these kinds of relationships learn how to deal with each other as real people, not as characters in films or books.

3

Agreements

No successful business can function without contracts. A legal contract is a statement of what each party wants from the other and which is negotiated and agreed by each. Legal action can be taken if it's broken, and the offending party can be called to account. It's not quite the same in relationships, in which the only legally binding contracts are related to marriage or parenthood. There are similarities though, and negotiating contracts in some relationships can be a good idea.

A contract gives you a basis for understanding each other. It sets some rules and allows you to be able to depend on each other to some extent. Some people balk at the idea of relationships having rules, but actually all relationships have them, it's just that they aren't usually recognized as such. How many times have you heard someone say, 'I don't treat people like that so why should they behave that way towards me?' or 'That's not playing fair'? This kind of comment shows the person is working by a set of rules, and believes the other person understands (or should understand) them.

In any relationship people want others to behave in a way which shows respect and acceptance of them, and conflicts and fights occur when the unwritten rules are broken. Have you ever said, 'If you really loved me, you would know what I want'? If the rules aren't explicit, how can people know how to keep them, even if they want to? If you expect others to be mind-readers about what you want, or believe, then you're in for disappointment. You could even find yourself accusing the other person of being uncaring because they don't instinctively know what to do or say to please you. Without direct requests and negotiations you run the risk of waiting for it all to equal. You'll do them a favour, or be nice, and they'll be good to you in return, or so you hope.

The 'You scratch my back and I'll scratch yours' idea is all very well, but the itch needs to be pointed out first. Some people miss this important factor but still keep score in their head of the number of favours they've done compared to how many they think they've received. If the score doesn't tally there's trouble. As far as the other person is concerned, it could seem like a storm that blows up from nowhere, since they have no ability to read the scorecard you are keeping.

It's likely that if you find yourself in conflict with someone it's because you don't have a clear contract. When people say things like, 'You said . . .', 'You promised . . .', 'You're not being fair', the real problem may be that there wasn't a clear agreement made in the first place. Contracts are not orders, they are agreements drawn up between *consenting* people. One person's assumption of the right way to do things is not an agreement.

A good relationship contract will arise from *wanting* to be with the other person, not *having* to be with them. This means that although you want to be together, you each have your own individuality, personality and are separate from each other. In this way you will form an alliance rather than create a dictatorship. A contract should be clearly stated and based on the understanding that you intend to keep it. You will always have the opportunity to renegotiate it if it isn't working or proves too restrictive.

It's no good striking a deal which begins with, 'Well, all right, if you insist . . .', or 'If that's the only way to keep you happy', or 'I don't have any choice'. They are all indications that the contract which follows is agreed under duress and will probably turn out unsatisfactorily. All the people involved in a contract should stand to gain something from it. This means it won't be one-sided. When it's clear to the other person you are interested in giving them as much as you're taking they can rest assured that you respect and care for them and aren't going to ride rough-shod over them.

Contracts can be made between teachers and pupils, parents and children, husbands and wives, lovers, friends, work colleagues — in fact any people who are sharing their lives or work together.

If you have a relationship in which there are constant arguments and battles of will, you might think of setting up a contract between you that would deal with some of the issues at stake.

Making a contract

There are six steps to making a contract:

Step 1: Think about what it is you want from the other person, and also what you are prepared to give.

Step 2: Write down the points you come up with. Make sure you're concentrating on specific and reasonable things. For instance, it's pointless wanting someone to change their personality for you — people only change when they choose to, not because someone else wants them to. Of course, if you are bigger or stronger than the other person, or have some real power over them, you may coerce them into changing their behaviour if they are afraid, but that is not a real change. The resentment they will feel as a result will make itself felt somehow at some time, and any relationship which depends on this kind of coercion will not in the long run be successful. You can, though, reasonably ask someone to change specific behaviour which would also be beneficial to them.

Step 3: Warn the person in advance that you're thinking about an issue and want to talk to them about it. Then they, too, can have a chance to think through what's wanted. You might say, for instance, 'There's something I've been wanting to say for some time. I haven't been happy about the way things are going between us and I'd like to talk about it when we meet on . . . to see if we can make things better'. In even the most intimate relationships you can make dates to talk about specific things. Be careful, though, not to use bribery: a quiet dinner for two can be a nice surprise, but if it comes with a sting in the tail — 'I've been nice to you, so you be agreeable to what I ask' — then the person may well feel they have been conned into an agreement. It's often better to make a direct arrangement to discuss anything of real seriousness and to make that the main purpose of the date. The intimate dinner, the carefully chosen gift, will be more appropriate after the agreement rather than being offered as an inducement.

Step 4: Make it clear you want to make a contract between you which is agreeable to both, and that you're not only interested in winning points.

Step 5: Take each point one at a time. Avoid confusing one issue with another. For instance, '. . . and while we're talking about this, what about your habit of being half-an-hour late. . . .' Also, avoid bringing up the distant past, '. . . and in 1983 you. . . .'

Step 6: Look and listen to each other. Make sure you hear the other person's response to you, and check you've understood it properly, e.g. 'I just want to make sure I've got it right. What you are suggesting is. . . .'

Contracts can be useful in all kinds of situations and problems. You could, for instance, draw up an agreement about time-keeping (for example, what time you come in, or unpunctuality), privacy (what you both expect to keep private), household chores (do you take it in turns or each have set tasks?), irritating behaviour (for example, nail biting or monopolizing the bathroom, or witholding physical affection).

Here is a sample contract between a son and his mother:

The son wanted	*The mother wanted*
To keep my room just as I like	Your room kept clean
To stay out at night as long as I like	You to be in by 11.00 pm
Not to keep having to explain what I'm doing or where I'm going	To know where you are

They discussed these things which had been the source of many rows and came up with the following agreements:

The son will clean his room at least once a week, and in return no-one else will go into it unless invited.

The son will be in by 11.00 pm on school nights, and stay out as long as he likes at the weekend.

Mother won't ask her son where he's been, but he will always give a phone number or address if he's going to be away all night.

More important than the actual agreements, each ended the discussion with a greater understanding of the other person. The son realized that his mother was genuinely concerned for him and not just trying to control him for the sake of it; the mother learned that her son was much more responsible than she had given him credit for.

Acceptance without judgement

People need to feel free to be themselves in a close relationship. If someone is upsetting you, then of course you have a right to tell them, and to ask them to behave differently — the same right as they have towards you. There is a difference, though, between wanting someone to change their behaviour towards you, and wanting them to *be* a different person — to have different beliefs, different preferences and so on. In relationships where people are expected to become someone different, when one is trying to mould the other to their own ideal, then trouble is in store. People who have trouble in their relationships often say things like, 'If you were different, everything would be OK'.

Blaming someone else for your own thoughts and feelings, dumping the responsibility in their court, merely paralyses you — if they won't change then you're stuck. If you accept that they are as they are, and that your reactions and feelings are your own, then you can change if you wish. This means that you may have to let go your wish to have an 'ideal' partner, friend, parent or child, and give up your efforts to make them into what is no more than a fantasy.

It may also mean that you give up your own need to be the perfect partner — the person who can get on with everyone. You need to accept your own wishes, values, and preferences and to understand that not everyone in the world will approve of or like you. There will be some people with whom you will not be able to maintain a good relationship, and it may be wiser to let them go rather than hold on in the hope that if you change enough they will stay with you.

Respect

Respect for yourself is not the same as conceit or arrogance. It means appreciating those things about yourself you're proud of as well as recognizing aspects you may wish to change. If you have respect for yourself you won't allow yourself to be walked over and abused. You will be aware and sensitive to what you are thinking and feeling, what you want and need, just as you will be sensitive to, and want to understand, what the other person is experiencing. You will have your share in any decisions, but you won't need to impose these at other people's expense.

In a growing relationship it's necessary for people to open themselves up by sharing their thoughts and feelings. This can't happen if there isn't mutual respect, a feeling that you both want to look after each other and contribute towards helping both of you develop and be happy.

Listening

Listening is an essential ingredient for making and keeping relationships. If you're a good listener, people will want to talk to you and your friendships will deepen. Those who don't listen turn off potential friends. They give the impression of someone who isn't interested in anyone but themselves. Non-listeners are also at a great disadvantage as they risk missing important information which might help them understand why people behave as they do. To please others the non-listener has to rely on guesses or mind-reading, and may well get it all wrong.

Listening is more than just being quiet when someone is talking, or waiting for them to stop so that you can say your twopenceworth. It's more than measuring what someone is saying to check whether you think it's right or wrong, whether you agree with it or not. That kind of listening is actually listening to yourself, not the other person at all. These are some of the kind of things you might hear from yourself which will drown out the other person:

'Look as if you're interested, then they'll like you.'

'Let them keep talking, it'll give you time to decide how to answer.'

'If you keep quiet, they won't realize how little you know.'

'How can you prove they're wrong'?

'Look out, they might be out to reject you.'

'If you don't listen they'll be hurt.'

'I wish they'd get to the point; I want to do something else!'

When you're really listening you will be intent on wanting to understand, wanting to help, or just enjoying what they are saying.

If you want to be a better listener, set yourself this task:

Choose someone who you would like to get on with better and next time you're talking together make yourself into a real listener. Clear your mind of your own concerns and concentrate only on what they're saying. Whenever they finish talking say something which shows you've understood or are trying to. For instance you could say, 'It sounds as if you enjoyed . . . though I'm not sure what you meant by. . . .' Check out what you've heard, especially if, to truly understand, you need a few things clarified. Only give your point of view once you've established you've understood and taken in what the other person has said.

After the conversation ask yourself:

How much do I understand his/her thoughts and feelings?

How much did I enjoy being with him/her?
What have I learned about him/her?
In what way did I help him/her?

Once you're willing to listen, and listen well, you'll be able to avoid some of the worst barriers to good communication.

The kind of barriers we mean include saying things like:

'You brought it on yourself — you've got no-one to blame but yourself.' (*Making judgement and offering no help at all*)

'You are insensitive and uncaring'; 'That is a terrible thing to do.' (*Negative criticism*)

'You're an idiot'; 'You can't be serious'; 'Well, that was clever, wasn't it!' 'Typical for a woman.' (*Putting down, sarcasm*)

'I can read you like a book'; 'I know just how your mind works.' (*Pretending you have a magic power which enables you to know what they're thinking*)

'You're such a good girl, I know you'll do the washing up'; 'You are so unselfish, I don't know how I'd manage without your help.' (*Bribing someone with praise so they will do what you want*)

'Shut up, and do it now'; 'I don't want to hear any reasons, just get on with it'; 'Do as I tell you.' (*Giving orders and taking no account of the other person's needs*)

'You do it — or else'; 'If you don't co-operate, I'll see you suffer.' (*Trying to control someone by making them afraid*)

'You mustn't split up, think of the children.' (*Moralizing and telling someone what they should do*)

'When did it happen? How did it happen? Why did you do it?' (*Firing questions, one after the other, like an inquisition*)

'If I were you, I'd . . .'; 'Why don't you . . .' (*Giving people advice based on what you would do if you were them*)

Direct communication

Imagine this scene:

Jenny: Do we have to go out to eat tonight?

Alan: Why, don't you feel like it?
Jenny: Well, it's just that we've been out every night this week.
Alan: Would you rather not go?
Jenny: Oh, no. Not if you want to.
Alan: What would you rather do?
Jenny: Oh, never mind. We'll go out.

Jenny is probably in for a miserable evening, as she's tired and would have preferred to stay at home and rest. As it is, Alan can't respond to her needs because he doesn't know what they are even though he has asked. Jenny won't say, but hopes he will read her mind and know why she wants to stay at home. It may be her way of trying to prove whether Alan really loves her, so if this is a typical conversation in their relationship it is easy to see how in time each will become dissatisfied with the other. Alan feeling manipulated and frustrated; Jenny feeling neglected and uncared for.

Communicating directly with people means telling them what you notice, what you think, what you feel and what you want.

What you notice: This means reporting what your senses tell you, without speculation or interpretation. For instance you may notice that someone is wearing a red dress; that they've got black hair. You may see a story about a train crash in the newspaper; you may experience heat or cold; hear a car coming or taste a spicy meal.

What you think: Thoughts are conclusions drawn from what you've experienced through your senses; judgements on whether something is good or bad; right or wrong. Beliefs, opinions, theories are all thoughts based on such judgements. For instance you may conclude that the red dress is much too bright for the occasion; that the hair is too short; that the train crash was due to the driver's incompetence. You may believe that faithfulness is necessary for a good marriage; you may have developed an opinion that too much sugar is bad for you; you may theorize from things you've been told or read that the behaviour of someone you know is due to his unhappy childhood.

What you feel: This is probably the most difficult thing to communicate. Sometimes people are afraid of emotion — their own and other people's. When we experience something strongly, we can feel hurt or disturbed in some way and this may be so unpleasant that we try to avoid it altogether. Some people learn early on in life that feelings are dangerous things. Parents are often scared by the strength of their children's emotions and may give out the message that it is somehow wrong for the child to feel so much. So excitement may be quashed in case it 'ends in tears' or crying may be discouraged as 'You'll soon get over it' or 'Only babies cry'.

If you don't take someone into your confidence about what pleases, annoys, frightens, saddens or excites you, then how can they respond to you with understanding. If you tell someone you've missed them they may give you a hug of reassurance. If you tell them you're angry that they didn't do the washing up then they'll know next time. If you tell them that you're getting anxious about an interview they can perhaps help you go over questions you may be asked or boost your ego in readiness.

What you want: No-one else knows what you want — they can guess, but they cannot know unless you tell them. You are the only person who knows you inside out, knows everything about you. However, you may have learnt that expressing your needs is wrong. Perhaps you were told, 'I want never gets!' or 'Don't be so selfish!' or 'Those that ask never get!' If those that asked never got then we'd have to learn to depend on the ability of others to know what we're thinking. We would then only be able to measure how much people really love us by how clairvoyant they were.

The other trap in thinking it's bad to ask for anything is to believe that we can ask if we become angry enough: 'You made me!' 'I shouldn't have to ask'. Asking for what you want directly can save a lot of beating around the bush, getting nowhere except becoming more frustrated and disappointed. If you want someone to stop arguing with you, ask them. If you want someone to help with the housework, ask. If you want to be given time to think, ask for it. Of course, asking doesn't necessarily mean you'll get what you want, it could lead to a refusal, a compromise or complete agreement. Whatever happens you will at least know where you stand and will be able to take responsibility for your own reactions, instead of having to depend totally on someone else to take responsibility for fulfilling your needs.

Good communication includes all these elements. If Jenny had given a complete message to Alan, she would have said something like:

'We've been out every night this week (observation) *and so many*

late nights mean that I'm tired now (thought). *I've enjoyed going out a lot, but I've got an important day ahead tomorrow at work and I'm anxious about being at my best for it* (feeling). *I'd really love to stay at home and have a lazy evening and an early night* (desire).'

This would have told Alan exactly what the situation was and what Jenny wanted, and he would have had more of a chance to respond positively than simply be left feeling confused.

Obviously not every situation warrants such attention. If you're asking someone the way, or buying a loaf of bread, the stranger you're talking to will not want to have a deep and meaningful discussion about your innermost feelings! If your boss asks you to do something, she will probably not appreciate a long speech detailing your emotional response! However, in relationships which matter and in which you are aiming for mutual understanding and care, try to express all four elements.

Getting into the habit of dealing with friends, colleagues and family this way should mean you know where you stand with them — and of course they will know where they stand with you. These relationships are likely to be less conflictive and disappointing than those in which the communication is indirect, and needs are only expressed covertly.

Remember, describe what you notice, say what you think and feel about it and ask for what you want.

A few more pointers in the line of direct communication are:

Be straight: Sometimes people avoid being direct because they're afraid of being laughed at or thought weak. They may also be anxious about the effect of their appearing to criticize someone by telling them about annoying traits. It isn't weak to tell people what you're feeling — in fact just the opposite. Cowards tend to run away, those with guts stick around to try to sort things out. As for giving offence, it's as well to remember that criticism needn't only be negative. Positive criticism can encourage someone to try again, or to change, rather than deflate them.

John's mother constantly nagged him about low marks he was getting at school. His marks went up and his mother stopped nagging him. But then she didn't say anything about his schoolwork, good or bad. He began to feel unappreciated and ignored. The message he was getting was that he only got attention when he did badly.

It is just as important to tell people when you are pleased with what they are doing as criticizing them when you aren't. If you are careful to do this, you will find that people will accept any criticism you make since they will realise that you are trying to help them rather than control them.

Be immediate: Don't delay in expressing what you want to say longer than is necessary. You can sit on angry and hurt feelings and even think you've hidden them from yourself, but they continue to smoulder away and will if left burst into flame at some unpredictable point. It's surprising how we find ways of getting our own back on people who have upset us: a sly comment, a sulk, indirect punishment of unspecified crimes. Sometimes we collect feelings without expressing them until we have enough stored up to feel we can justify an explosion of anger and have a row or become overwhelmed with grief, and burst into tears. Some people allow things to fester for years, and then when they do have a row resurrect all the old grievances: '. . . and I remember three years ago when you left me waiting for half an hour, and not only that but you borrowed a book last year which you haven't returned and. . . .' Of course, by the time such stored grievances are expressed there may be no way to put them right.

Swallowed anger or hurt can turn inward and begin eating away at the person's core of self-esteem and security. It may turn into depression so that the person, and those closest to them, suffer as a result. The other destructive effect is when those feelings which aren't expressed to those directly involved are vented on innocent victims — shop assistants, people on the end of the telephone, someone who just happens to get in your way, employees. It isn't fair on those who catch the full force of your anger, since they can do nothing about the situation which causes it. It doesn't help you much either, except as a very short-term way of getting some relief from the tension. It could also add to a burden of guilt.

The advantage of dealing immediately with something which has upset you is that if the person you're dealing with learns quickly what you need, they are more likely to be able to respond to you. It also makes you more real, more human. There is something almost robot-like about people who don't express feelings, who always remain calm and unmoved.

Be clear: There are many ways in which we can muddy our communication. One example is asking questions instead of stating an opinion. For instance, a wife might say to her husband, 'Do you really want to do that overtime?', instead of what she really means, which is, 'I'm afraid that if you take on this extra work, I'll see even less of you and I'm worried our relationship will suffer.' Meanwhile her husband may wonder whether his wife means that they don't need the money, or is worried that he's trying to avoid her, or saying he should really be putting up shelves at home.

Other people may well guess when you're hiding things from them, especially if what you're actually saying doesn't match your body language and tone of voice. If you ask someone how they feel and they answer, 'I'm fine, thank you' and you notice their body is tense, brow furrowed and hands clenched, it just doesn't add up and you'll be left wondering what may be troubling them. Saying one thing on the surface when the body is telling another tale can only lead to confusion. Of course, it's not only the body which can contradict the spoken word, it's possible to give double messages in the same breath. Examples of this are: 'Of course I love you. I just wish you would behave differently sometimes', or 'Go ahead, have a good time. I suppose I'll be all right here on my own.'

So, to summarize, healthy relationships are ones in which the people concerned will show mutual respect and acceptance, will listen to each other and share their thoughts and feelings. Easier said than done, because we all have our own particular hang-ups, but if you are willing to work on our suggestions you will be bound to reap rewards.

4

Will it last?

Love can open doors. Being part of a couple does offer things we cannot get on our own, such as companionship, sharing needs, emotional and practical support. Most people during their lives get involved in one or more such relationships, or try very hard to do so. In this chapter we'll look at making couples work for both people, and some of the obstacles in the way of that.

Whilst 'coupledom' can provide the opportunity for certain things, it's also important to accept that having a partner is not the be all and end all of life. Some people never make such commitments, or make them but don't keep them. Others are left by a loved one, through choice or death. In our society, in which there is a pressure for everyone to be like everyone else, a couple sometimes seems to be more valued than a single person. You have only to listen to a widow or widower, or a newly divorced person, describing how their friends suddenly seem embarrassed by them — how they're never invited to social events at which they were once regulars and how if they do go they feel the odd one out. Listen, too, to teenagers who feel odd because they haven't had a girl- or boyfriend, or they haven't got a steady and their friends have. They all seem to believe that it's a sign of failure to be without a partner. If you want to share your life with someone in a permanent relationship, then of course it's right for you to keep your eyes open for such a person. You should be sure though that you want this because it's right for you, and not because it shows you can keep the 'rules'. If you are happier on your own you are not abnormal.

So while in this book we're mostly dealing with couples, we don't want to give the impression that people who aren't paired off are abnormal or failures. Being on your own can have its own rewards, pressures and pain, as can being a couple or a family.

Wouldn't life be simple if it were possible to give a blueprint for building relationships? Unfortunately it isn't. Nor is it possible to give guarantees that any relationship you get involved in will be successful. All you can do is maximize your chances, and in this chapter are guidelines and pointers to help you avoid common obstacles.

A major obstacle is the fact that two people come to a

relationship with two different sets of expectations. Both will have had different experiences in life, and will have been influenced by different things or people. One person's idea of the 'right' way to love may be at variance with the other's thinking. What one person finds easy to express the other may not. One may be physically demonstrative, the other not. Some people love candlelight and roses whilst others are happier watching stock-car racing. Some people plunge quickly and deeply into a relationship, while others prefer to have a number of less passionate and more gentle friendships out of which love may arise. Some people want to devote all their time to one relationship. Others feel happier dividing their time with other interests. Some people believe that sex is the ultimate expression of loving someone and will postpone making love until they know each other well or are married. Others want sex to be part of close relationships from the start. There are those who deliberately pick certain partners for their advantages and disadvantages, and others who believe that this is cold and calculating and act according to their intuition.

None of these styles of loving is 'right' or 'wrong', but they are different. You can imagine the trouble two lovers could have if they have different approaches.

If you'd like to clarify your own style, here is an exercise that might help you:

Think of a story that you loved when you were a child — a fairy story for instance. Write the story as you remember it, or speak it into a tape recorder. Don't worry about whether it's right or wrong, or about bits you can't remember at all, just recount what you can remember.

Then answer these questions about the story you have just told:

(a) Who's the hero, and what are the main features of his character.

(b) Who is the heroine, and what are the main features of her character?

(c) Who is the villain, and what are the main features of their character?

(d) With whom do you identify most?

(e) Is there anything in the character or behaviour of this person that reminds you of yourself?

(f) How does the story end?

(g) How does the character with whom you identify end up?
(h) Is there anything similar to how you see your life progressing?
(i) Is there some way in which you would prefer the story to end?
(j) What would have to happen in order for this to happen?

A relationship is like a journey, and like most journeys it begins with a great deal of excitement and hope. Those caught in the romance trap hang onto the belief that their journey will be smooth and consistently pleasurable, ending in some wonderful sunset with the music swelling and engulfing the happy couple. Disappointingly, the actual experience of most people doesn't tally with that romantic vision. In reality, when two people get together there will be times when they feel very close to each other, times when they get on each other's nerves or argue, and times when they seem to move away from each other. Many relationships move through recognizable stages.

Getting together

This is the time when lovers only have eyes for each other. If apart for long they pine, as they don't like to be physically separated. The whole focus of their attention is their relationship, and for a while everything takes second place to that. A great deal of intimacy is developed between the pair and they feel 'in love' — onlookers may say 'lovesick'. During this period in their relationship a couple create a kind of closed system into which it's very difficult for others to intrude. It's an exciting time, when each wants to please and be pleased by the other. Any differences in their view of the world or how they cope with life will be glossed over, or not even noticed.

Being together

The overwhelming passion fades. If the couple continue to feel good about sharing their lives and are willing and able to give each other support then the first stage has been successfully negotiated. 'In love' becomes love.

In this second phase of a relationship the couple will still want to create a life together, sometimes at the expense of their individual needs and preferences. They are no longer two separate people who get together, they establish themselves as a new unit. A couple who choose to live together may spend a lot of energy jointly creating their home — nest-building as it's sometimes called. They're also likely to spend most of their social life with other 'couples'. They're establishing themselves as a new unit.

Those who mistook passion for compatibility will hit a rocky ride at this point. They may continue to live together, but it will be a time of considerable conflict with each suffering the pain of shattered dreams. They may break up or they may develop a pattern of avoiding conflicts, brushing problems under the carpet. At this point some couples have children to try and bridge the gap between them. Their mutual desire to care for a child may indeed allow them to do this, but at some cost — to themselves in the long run, and certainly to the child who bears the responsibility for keeping the parents together. For others, though, their very attempt to bridge the gap actually forces them apart when the weight of childcaring and the demands of a third person take hold.

Moving apart

At some stage in their shared journey, perhaps after months or even many years, the partners may begin to feel the need to express their individuality, to be their own person again and not simply someone's 'other half'. This need for one or both to loosen the ties, or to develop parts of their personality or skills previously neglected could assert itself at any time. Other changes may precipitate this separating — for instance, it's common for a couple to re-examine their own roles in life when the children in a family grow up. Then the parents are left with more time on their hands to do things and to think about what they've got out of their lives so far, and what they still want. The shift could come much earlier, though.

Couples who have faced and worked through their difficulties, will negotiate this stage with fewer conflicts and crises than partners who have avoided any potential clashes. That's not to say there won't be any crises, but they'll have learnt how to negotiate with each other. They'll also feel more able to understand the other partner's need to develop as an individual without seeing it as a fundamental threat to the relationship.

On the other hand, some couples cover up problems in their relationship by being constantly busy. Work or hobbies may become all-absorbing or child-rearing may be the all-important activity. When the work is no longer there, perhaps as a result of redundancy or retirement, or when the children leave home, the cracks emerge and can no longer be avoided.

Staying together

Reaching the last leg of a journey can be very satisfying. If a couple have worked through their problems successfully an increasing sense of closeness and harmony often develops. A sense of calm and acceptance prevails. It can be almost as if they are 'in love' again and some people in their later years show a closer sense of togetherness than younger people. But, like the preceeding stages, if previous storms haven't been weathered, a break-up may become inevitable or an uneasy truce called.

There's no guarantee your relationships will follow this pattern rigidly, but it's a rough sketch of common experience. To complicate matters, though, no two people will go through this cycle at precisely the same rate. Partners can get out of step with each other, so you cannot expect your lover to remain in perfect tune with you, however harmonious everything seemed at the beginning.

Not realizing this natural progression in relationships, some young or 'new' couples may panic when one partner suddenly wants to go out on his or her own, or change the way the partnership has been. This desire for change may be quite healthy, but the panic of being left behind can make someone clingy, and make change very difficult to achieve. If you're in a relationship, and though being quite contented want to explore a bit more of yourself, do explain why to your partner — that it's not their fault, and you do still care for them. If the boot is on the other foot, and your partner is requesting more freedom, then do remember not to make catastrophies out of simple requests. A night out with the girls does *not* mean she's leaving you! In fact she may come back refreshed and keen to see you after the 'separation'.

If either individual's personal needs are squashed by the 'a couple must do everything together' mentality, then trouble will almost inevitably strike.

Although many people find that in their later years they feel closer to the partner with whom they've shared life's ups and downs, if one partner has been bottling feelings up for 30 years the needs and desires they've been covering up may suddenly bubble to the surface with such force they can no longer be ignored. Take Jennifer for example.

Jennifer married at 19 and soon after had her first baby. She raised five children and took pride in being what she thought of as a 'model wife and mother', looking after her husband, keeping the house spotless, and making sure the children had every opportunity to fulfil their ambitions.

When the youngest child left home to go to university, Jennifer became very depressed. On the face of it there was no reason for the depression — she had been extremely successful in her role as wife and mother, and stretching ahead of her was the possibility to take life a bit easier. She dabbled with painting and photography, hobbies which she had enjoyed for many years, but the depression continued. She joined a self-help group in which she had the opportunity to explore her own feelings with other people who were also feeling dissatisfied. She realized that ever since her marriage she had organized her life to fit in with other people — her husband and her children. She had been too busy to identify and fulfil her own needs.

Jennifer is at the moment a full-time student — she won a mature student place at University. Her husband resented her decision, and has left home to live with another woman. Jennifer certainly didn't want that to be one of the consequences of her choice, but knows she doesn't want to give up this new life which allows her to be her own person for the first time in her life.

Most relationships seem to follow a pattern of moving together and apart as different phases of development occur, but don't depend on your partner to follow your own pattern of development at exactly the same rate. Surviving the problems such changes may bring will depend on the ability and willingness of both of you to confront difficulties rather than avoid them.

The ability to change, to evolve, is the crucial sign of life in any organism, and people who are able to adapt to change will feel that their relationship is alive and dynamic. If there are no changes, the relationship will, sooner or later, feel stale and monotonous, and the couple will get bored.

In the beginning of any relationship both people are adapting to each other and to a new lifestyle, so there's a feeling of excitement. However the rate of change inevitably slows down as they come to know what to expect from each other, and although there can still be surprises in store, it's only in the romantic world that relationships remain on the same high after the initial excitement. Sometimes this reality comes as a shock to people. An example of this is what's called post-honeymoon blues.

Most cultures mark the occasion of two people making a

commitment to each other with a ceremony of some kind, religious or otherwise, and in our culture we also tend to celebrate the event with a party or a holiday, or both. For most couples this is a time of enormous excitement and hope — the future seems to stretch ahead full of happiness, and no problem is too great to be solved. Sooner or later real life intrudes. A monotonous job is no less monotonous now that the person is married or living with another, household chores still have to be done, problems the couple may have had beforehand haven't magically disappeared, dominating parents haven't become paragons of non-interference, and so on.

Most couples come to terms with this, but those who expected life to cruise along because they'd found a partner may convince themselves that something has gone wrong. They may dream about how wonderful things used to be, or blame their partner for not staying the same. Their conversation becomes peppered with accusations beginning with phrases like 'Do you remember when . . .', 'You always used to . . .' Eventually this disillusionment will cause the relationship to break up or settle into an uneasy alliance where each feels disappointed and unfulfilled.

It may seem as if we're hammering this point home, but it's important to accept that change is inevitable, that you and your partner will change as both your lives develop, separately and together. You will age, present priorities may lose their urgency and others take their place, you will each have experiences which may alter your outlook on life, and so on.

Partners changing at different rates can create conflict, particularly if each one is depending on the other to remain the same. To be able to deal positively with this they need to see that conflict is evidence that a relationship is alive. For relationships to survive each needs to allow the other to be a whole person, not one half of a whole. To quote Kahlil Gibran's *The Prophet*:

> Give your hearts, but not into each other's keeping
> For only the hand of Life can contain your hearts,
> And stand together yet not too near together:
> For the pillars of the temple stand apart,
> And the oak tree and the cypress grow not in each other's shadow.

Barriers to Survival

People will only stay contented and together for a long time if they're willing to include their differences, and accept them rather than avoid them or try to manipulate the other person into changing. None of this is easy — living with another person can be very difficult and many relationships don't survive the stresses and strains. We'll now move on to explore some of those stresses which could be created by some of the beliefs which each of us may carry into a relationship. Each belief creates a barrier which stands in the way of moving through the difficulties.

Barrier One

'Silence is Golden'

In a relationship this just isn't true. Not talking about something can seem like an easy way out. It's not. If you're going to work constructively through inevitable changes then they will need discussing and negotiating, and feelings will need to be understood. Those may be painful feelings so it sometimes seems simpler all round to avoid such issues. But things don't disappear, problems don't just go away because they're not talked about — often quite the reverse.

Listen to Geraldine talking to a marriage guidance counsellor:

> 'He just ignores me. Every time I say I want to talk about how our relationship is going he buries himself in a newspaper — or says he must fix the car or says I shouldn't get so serious. Sometimes I get really desperate and shout and cry, but he just won't respond. I wouldn't mind if he got angry back at me, at least that would be better than no response at all. I don't think he cares for me at all.'

Silence can be a more vicious weapon than words. The person who refuses to respond to a partner's needs for communication, refuses to give any feedback, is often using their silence as a way of controlling the other. Although on the surface it may look as if Geraldine is controlling her husband, because she makes more noise than he does, and may be accused of nagging, in fact it is he who is in control. She feels driven to extreme behaviour in order to get any response at all from him.

Some people are frightened that talking about something will only make things worse. It may for a while. Bringing a problem out into the open can make things feel considerably more unpleasant than the superficially pleasant cover-up there might have been before. So, what possible good can talking do?

By pretending problems don't exist, and by avoiding the issues — so effectively avoiding each other — individuals grow apart. Unfortunately conflicts which are ignored rarely disappear but remain as irritants. For the person whose wants are unmet, those desires become more and more important, perhaps eventually out of all proportion. This leads inevitably to resentment simmering under a pseudo-harmony.

Finding the words can be difficult. It is hard to talk about our innermost feelings — for one thing the English language is notably lacking in vocabulary which expresses feelings. Fumbling for words in an attempt to express ourselves accurately, and searching too hard for just the right word or phrase can induce a kind of verbal paralysis. Since the 'right' word probably doesn't exist, try not to get tongue-tied, speak your mind and let the *way* you say things help you out.

The stiff-upper-lip brigade have a lot to answer for. All those John Wayne movies, where the hero was the strong, silent saviour of the town, fighting off the baddies and winning the heroine, all without moving a facial muscle, are examples of how our culture values that kind of behaviour. Of course it's complete nonsense that only the weak show how they feel and that the strongest are those who go through life without shedding a tear. Strong people are ones who can form healthy friendships and relationships. Healthy relationships are based on people sharing themselves and their experiences. Our emotional responses are an integral part of us, and to hide them from people we share our lives with means denying the relationship an essential part of ourselves.

Some feelings are hard to express: loneliness, jealousy, inadequacy, for instance. It's tempting to fall back on familiar phrases like 'It's your fault I feel like this' or 'You make me so angry'. It's important to accept that how you feel is something *you* are responsible for. Of course the other person is responsible for what they are or are not doing, and you have a right to hold them responsible and to ask them to change their behaviour. The one thing they aren't responsible for, though, is how you react to such behaviour. That is something that is created by your own mind and body, and will be a result of your own perception of the world, your own physical and mental state at the time, and the role you've developed for yourself.

The best solution to all of this is to try and be honest and communicate what you're thinking and feeling. You may feel daft or self-conscious if this is something you're unused to, but in time, with practice, you'll find it quite natural and beneficial.

Of course you can talk too much. You don't need to analyse why you or your partner chose cornflakes for breakfast when they normally prefer toast, but if you find you're mulling on something, or are irritated by particular behaviour, it's probably best to get it off your chest. It's better in the long run to share your feelings with your partner, both 'good' and 'bad' as immediately as practical. That way small resentments won't collect together and build up into an enormous explosive anger which hits the unsuspecting partner like a bolt from the blue.

When it feels as if conflict is in the air it can be handy to have a formula for trying to sort out problems rather than retire into entrenched positions ready to declare war.

The five Rs

1. Reflect Before you do anything, think about what you want to say, particularly if you want to criticize. It's very tempting to believe that if someone doesn't behave the way we want them to that we have the right to punish or coerce them. Criticizing others to exact some sort of revenge, or in order to force them to behave differently, usually fails in the long run. If the other person is afraid of you then they may well change their behaviour towards you, but you will lose their long-term co-operation and be treated in a very guarded fashion. So try to be sure that your main motives in saying your piece are to help educate or protect the other, or to solve a problem that you both have. If you hang on to these as your main motives then your attempts at plain speaking are far more likely to have positive results.

2. Report Once you've sorted out your motives and decided whether or not to go ahead, then reporting means saying exactly what is happening. Be as specific and objective as possible and avoid generalizations such as 'You always . . .', 'You never . . .', 'You're so thoughtless . . .' Instead describe just what you notice and talk about specific actions or events, such as 'You were an hour late . . .', 'When you interrupt me before I finish the sentence . . .' This is important because if you weigh in with very general and personal criticisms the other person will feel attacked, and get defensive. As one of the commonest forms of defence is attack, you can see how easily this could turn into a destructive battle. The person you are talking to is less likely to feel got at if you concentrate on specific events or issues rather than attacking them personally.

You can start off by easing yourself in with phrases like 'I'd like to discuss something with you now', 'I know I've never said this before, but I really do want to tell you. . .', 'I've noticed that . . .'

3. Relate Tell someone how their behaviour affects you, the emotional impact it has. You can do this by saying 'I feel . . .' — naming whatever feelings you experience, and then talk about any thoughts you have about it. Don't make the first focus your bad feelings, instead concentrate on the effects of actions — for example 'I think your behaviour and my reaction to it are hindering our relationship' is better than 'I think you're selfish and thoughtless and you make me extremely angry'. 'I feel insignificant when you criticize me in public' is preferable to 'I hate it when you . . .'

4. Request Ask for what you'd like to be different, and how. Make sure that your request is reasonable and within the power of the other person to give. Remember that you have a right to ask for whatever you want from someone, and they have exactly the same right to say yes or no. If you don't ask, though, it could be difficult, if not impossible, for them to know what will please you.

Try not to fall into the 'mind-reading' trap — believing that if the other person loved you enough they would instinctively give you what you wanted without you having to ask. You might wait an awfully long and disappointing time, while, if you asked, the other person might happily give you what you want. Even if they refuse, you at least know where you stand.

Avoid demanding — people often resist demands, not because they are unreasonable or impossible, but because no-one likes being pushed around! 'I'd prefer it if you waited until I'd finished what I have to say before telling me what you think' is preferable to 'Shut up until I've finished'. 'I'd really like to talk about how we can improve things between us' is preferable to 'We must talk about . . .'

Sometimes at this request stage you can negotiate a deal—'I'll do this for you, if you'll do that for me'.

5. ***Results*** Spell out the positive consequences you foresee from the change you want. People are more likely to co-operate with you if they know the reasoning and logic behind your request. Otherwise they might think you're just trying to manipulate them to show you're the boss. So, in rounding off saying your piece you could say something like 'I think I'll feel less defensive, and won't need to argue so much' or 'I won't feel you're out to get one over on me all the time'.

It's also wise to look at a negative result, when the person doesn't want to co-operate, and what you'll do about that. Unfortunately there's no golden rule which says that just because your request is reasonable the other person must agree to do what you want! If you find yourself in a position where either the other person breaks their part of an agreement, or refuses to change their behaviour, then you have some decisions to make.

You have several options. You can decide to live with them as they are because overall the good points about them outweigh the bad. You can decide to leave them because you don't want to be with someone who refuses to treat you seriously enough to consider or respond to your wants. You may decide that you don't want to leave them because you don't have the strength or resources to manage on your own, in which case you will have to begin working out ways of coping as well as possible with the situation, remembering you've chosen that path.

Whether or not you tell someone what you'll do if they turn down your request is up to you. It would be manipulative to use threats, but on the other hand if you know there is some action you will take it would be unfair to withold vital information. Don't bluff though, because if the other person calls your bluff and you back down then you run the risk of them never taking you seriously again.

The five Rs formula — Reflect, Report, Relate, Request and Results — will help you to determine your needs and rights, propose a resolution and, if necessary, to negotiate. Breaking it down this way means you may be able to think more clearly about what end result you want from a conflict, and why, and what you're prepared to do about it.

All this requires preparation and planning. You need to think about it. Though it might seem to make it rather academic, it may help to write out your 'script' for the talk beforehand. Writing things down can help clarify your own thoughts and feelings, and if it's clear in your own mind you can launch into a difficult conversation with a bit more confidence. It may also help you avoid emotional outbursts which you'd come to regret. Writing it all down will also mean you can review how well you did compared to your plan. The formula itself cannot guarantee success, and if you're not used to this kind of direct speaking you may find it doesn't go exactly as planned. Instead of criticizing yourself for failing, you will be able to match what you wanted to say against what actually happened. That will help you learn to be more effective next time.

Here are some examples of how people have used this idea.

> Joan gave her husband a lift to the station every morning. She found this inconvenient for a number of reasons, and wanted to change the arrangement. She had brought this up a few times, but on each occasion John would express surprise that she felt so strongly about what seemed to be a trivial matter, and she would respond by feeling guilty and dropping the subject.

This is the '5R' script she wrote:

Reflect: I know John expects me to drive him to the station every morning. When I started to do it I really enjoyed being able to help and please him in that way. I wasn't working myself and I loved starting the morning with him. Now my situation is different, and I want him to acknowledge that it's no longer a pleasure but a problem.

Report: John, I'd like to discuss my giving you a lift each morning. I know I've brought this up before, but it's still a problem for me and I'd like to talk it over again. I've been driving you each morning, and up till a few months ago I enjoyed it. Since then I've started work, and my office is in the opposite direction.

Relate: I feel put upon because you take it for granted that I'll carry on with this even though my situation has changed. Taking you to the station means I'm often late through being caught in the High Street traffic, which I could avoid if I went straight to my office.

Request: I'd prefer you to walk, or take the bus — or if you don't want to do that, to discuss the possibility of getting another car. If you decide to walk, I'm willing to give you a lift when the weather is very bad.

Result: This way I won't feel so resentful at being taken for granted and won't be so worried each morning that I'll be late.

When Joan approached John with this he was momentarily taken aback by the fact that she obviously had thought through what she wanted, and wasn't nagging or getting at him. This in turn meant he couldn't discount her as easily as he had in the past, and so had to consider her suggestions. In fact, he decided to walk the fifteen minutes to the station, agreeing with Joan to discuss it again if it became a problem for him.

Many people feel resentful about being taken for granted, or about having their own time used up in doing 'favours' for other people. Sometimes, like Joan, they start doing something as a pleasure or a treat and later find they're expected to go on doing it forever, and then it becomes a burden. Most of us enjoy helping others, but we dislike being taken advantage of or having excessive demands made on us. Saying, 'No, I no longer want to do this' or 'No, I want to spend my time/money/abilities some other way' may seem too embarrassing or frightening. Without tackling the problem, though, it simply means a build-up of more and more resentment.

Here is another example of a '5R' script.

Andy's partner is given to sulking on occasions when she doesn't get what she wants.

Reflect: Frances frequently acts as if she's angry with me, but won't answer me when I ask her what's wrong. She just looks at me as if she wishes looks could kill. I am increasingly irritated with this behaviour. I'm sure she's unhappy about something, but if I don't know what it is, I can't do anything about it. I want to continue living with her, but not like this.

Report: You just looked at me as if you were very angry with me. When I asked you what was the matter, you shrugged and looked away from me.

Relate: I feel very unhappy when you're silent. I'm worried that I'm upsetting you, and feel helpless because I don't know what to do about it. I want to consider your feelings, and your wants, but I don't know how.

Request: I'd like you to tell me directly when I've said or done something which hurts or angers you, and to tell me what you want me to do instead. We could take some time now, or decide a time, to talk things over. Will you agree to that?

Result: If we do this, I'll make every effort to change in the way you want, or work out a compromise with you. If you're unwilling to work this out, I'll no longer worry about improving our relationship.

Andy did have a conversation with Frances along those lines, but it was a difficult and entrenched problem, and it took quite a few attempts to reassure Frances that Andy genuinely wanted to solve the problem, and not control her. When they did begin talking openly Frances told Andy about some of his behaviour which upset her. For instance, he often spent time playing with his computer, so cutting back on the time they had together. She hadn't mentioned it before because she didn't know how, and was afraid he'd get angry. However, she wasn't able to hide her own strong feelings entirely, and so her silence added to the tensions.

This is an example of how two people, both feeling unhappy, can believe that the other is entirely to blame. In fact, as you can see with Frances and Andy, each carries some responsibility for the situation. It was only by talking that they were able to begin to understand what was going on between them. Assuming that the people involved want to continue together, this understanding will help them make the changes which will enable them to be happier with each other.

Here's an exercise for practice:
Think of a real situation in your life at the moment where you're avoiding telling or asking someone something. It could be asking for help or information, protesting about annoying habits, resisting unjust criticism, establishing your independence, saying no to unreasonable demands, dealing with sulking, and so on.

Write down what you've said (or not said) about it in the past.

Now write the following sentences, filling in the gaps with your own situation:
'I've noticed that you . . . (describe exactly what the other person

> does). *What happens in response to that is that I feel . . .* (describe what you're feeling — angry, sad, frightened, frustrated, etc.), *and I think that . . .* (describe any of your personal beliefs or values associated with it). *I'd prefer . . .* (state in specific terms exactly what you want), *because then . . .* (spell out the result).

One word of warning about all this. Obviously what we've said so far is that good relationships need open, direct communication. But it is possible to talk too much. Take for instance what happens between Caroline and Julian:

> They've agreed to be open with each other, and both take this very seriously. This means they make every minor disagreement, every small dissatisfaction, an opportunity to re-evaluate their relationship completely. Nothing is allowed to pass — everything is seen as an important symbol of what is happening between them.
>
> This has led to their being able to talk about little else. Every conversation between them is 'deep and meaningful', and this of course is very wearing and sometimes even boring! They both have begun to go back on their decision to tell each other everything, and as a result each is beginning to feel quilty and resentful, since it's sometimes easier to say nothing than to start another session in which each has to reveal their innermost thoughts and feelings.
>
> Unless Caroline and Julian come to realize that there needs to be some boundary established between them about what is and is not appropriate they will eventually split up.

Knowing when to talk and when to keep quiet can be difficult. One thing to remember is that whether or not you're saying anything with your words, you are always communicating. Messages are given out by tone of voice, by gestures and body language. The most valuable communication may be when you comfort or reassure your partner by putting your arm around them, or stroking their hair.

Check with your partner that the messages you intend to give are actually the ones they receive. Ask them to tell you what they think you're asking for. This will allow any misunderstandings to be cleared up before they grow into major and unnecessary grievances.

An example of where talking might be counter-productive is the confessing of an affair. Research into marital relationships shows that many married men and women have extra-marital relations at some point in their marriage. Whatever the motive for an affair, the result of discovery or confession is often the same. Strong feelings are aroused — jealousy, competitiveness, fear, anger, and so on. Many partnerships don't survive the discovery of infidelity.

Infidelity can carry an excitement which may be lacking in a long-term relationship, since affairs are usually unaffected by the more mundane yet necessary elements of everyday life. Because they are somehow 'unreal', affairs don't usually get beyond the first phase of a relationship, where the intensity of mutual attraction is all that matters. Passion rules this situation which is why sometimes people can be fooled into believing this new 'love' is more meaningful and significant than the original relationship. It may be, but perhaps when the passionate phase passes and the mists over your eyes clear they may view rather differently what they see.

Because such strong feelings are triggered off by this situation, it can be difficult for a couple to deal with the problem. There is often a strong temptation to 'confess', even after the event is well over, but this needs thinking about. Many such confessions are given in order that the 'guilty' party can be pardoned and approved of rather than being a real attempt at openness. Sometimes the partner who had the wandering eye may actually want to be 'punished' so that they no longer need feel guilty. Other confessions may be made as a way of forcing the end of an affair, giving a reason for it other than a change of heart.

Two-timing can kill a relationship — that's a fact. Even a passing passion can destroy the long built-up trust which must be part of a one-to-one relationship. Such passions do happen though. Once they have, there's no rule about whether it's always right or wrong to tell all. If you are in this position it may be wise to consider your motives before you reveal the facts. It may be that ending the affair and dealing with your own feelings about it is the most constructive thing to be done rather than actually burdening your long-term partner.

You may not wish to have an exclusive relationship with one person. If you don't then it's imperative you make that clear. Problems arise when one person believes they have an agreement including faithfulness when that's not how it is at all. Most people do prefer monogamy (one exclusive partner), and most religions and cultures preach it. There are obvious health considerations as well as the fact that sexual jealousy is extremely hard to overcome and deep intimacy difficult to sustain with more than one person.

Barrier Two

'Don't get too close'

Long-term relationships give us the opportunity to experience emotional intimacy, but that can be frightening. Often our communication with other people is on a pretty superficial level. If you meet someone in the street, you might as you pass them say 'Hello, how are you?' and they'll probably reply 'Fine thanks, how are you?'. It's the kind of conversation which takes place while the people involved are really thinking about something else. It's the sort of ritual that happens over and over again, and although there is some contact, it's not of a very lasting kind.

It's even perfectly possible to have long conversations with people but make no real contact with them. Comparing notes about cars, holidays or the latest fashions, grumbling about how awful 'it all' is, criticizing the education system, looney lefties, or rabid righties. All these are pastimes where the people talk a lot, but don't actually share much of themselves.

Intimacy is the kind of contact in which the people concerned feel able to be themselves, that they don't have to put on a show or pretend to be other than they are. In this kind of contact you know you'll be accepted 'warts and all' and the other person doesn't need to change in order to be acceptable to you. You'll share as much of your innermost thoughts and feelings as you want to, and will accept the other person in just the same way.

Intimacy is a frightening prospect for many people, because as we get closer to someone the fear of being rejected by them becomes greater. For some people this fear is so great that they won't allow themselves to get close to anyone in the first place, as a way of protecting themselves from getting hurt.

The psychologist Eric Berne, in his book *Games People Play* describes the destructive patterns of behaviour that people often develop as a way of avoiding intimacy. The patterns that he calls games are repetitive; once started they follow an inevitable course, usually ending with everyone involved feeling rotten. Games happen when people are saying or doing one thing whilst actually meaning something else.

He describes a game called 'Rapo' in which one person engages in titillating, flirtatious behaviour and when the other person responds by making some move towards them, they become indignant and say something like 'How dare you treat me like that!' In this game the 'seducer' is able to prove his or her power without engaging in actual intimacy with another.

Then there's the fairly common family game called 'Uproar'. A possible scenario is: husband comes home from work and finds fault with wife (the dinner isn't ready, or the kids' toys are on the floor). Wife becomes angry and shouts or cries. Their voices rise and the argument becomes more acute. This game nearly always ends with a slammed door! Either husband leaves for the pub, or the wife rushes out to have a good cry with a friend, or both retire to different rooms. At no time have either of them really talked about their true feelings towards each other, or expressed their wants in such a way that the other could respond positively.

> Helen and Emma play a game called 'Corner'. Helen suggests that they go to the cinema, and Emma agrees. Then in the course of conversation, Helen mentions that their flat needs decorating. This angers Emma, because she has recently been made redundant, and is no longer able to contribute as much as before to their shared budget. Helen, of course, knows this, but has somehow 'forgotten'. Helen takes offence at Emma's anger and says if that's how she feels, she no longer wants to go to the film.
>
> This game has several possible endings: neither go to the film and stay at home with Helen righteously indignant and Emma angry and resentful; Helen goes to the film alone; Emma goes to the film alone; they both go to the cinema, but neither enjoy it.

The 'corner' game is one in which someone is put into a position of being seen as unreasonable, and responsible for the other's problems. In the case of Helen and Emma neither is asking for what they want from the other. Helen wants to be shown appreciation for how hard she works, and Emma wants to be reassured that she is still cared for despite her feelings of failure at not being able to contribute materially as before.

There's one game that's very familiar to counsellors. It's called the 'Courtroom'. Played with a husband and wife it might go like this. The husband begins plaintively — 'I must tell you what she did last week. She forgot . . .'. The wife defends herself — 'That's not how it was. This is what really happened . . .'. The husband then adds — 'I'm glad that you can hear both sides of the story'. Now the counsellor (or friend/priest/doctor/health visitor/social worker, or whoever is playing the role of 'Judge') is meant to say wisely, 'Well, on hearing you both, this is what I think you should do'.

The purpose behind this game is to offload on someone else the responsibility for deciding who is right. Any friend or counsellor who finds themselves a participant in this drama would be much wiser to put the responsibility and decisions back where they belong, with the couple. In doing so, though, it's also useful to make them aware of the game they are playing and how, by side-tracking into that courtroom drama, they're avoiding tackling their real differences. There's also the bonus that if a couple settle the differences between them then they'll be less likely to contest the 'judgement' and appeal against the outsider's ruling.

Ironically, people who are afraid of intimacy may opt for a lifestyle full of relationships.

> Alan seemed to enjoy a life in which he had many sexual relationships, although from time to time he experienced deep depressions. On talking to a therapist, he admitted 'I really would like to settle down with someone special. I like all the people I go out with, but I can't seem to get really close to anyone.' The therapist pointed out that his casual lifestyle didn't actually allow him to get to know anyone very well, each relationship served to distract him from intimate contact rather than allow it to develop.

Game players avoid intimacy through fear. They may believe that allowing themselves to become dependent on someone else is a sign of weakness, or that they'll lose their ability to cope on their own. They may fear that if they allow someone else too close into their world they'll be overwhelmed, that the other person will become too dependent on them. Instead of expressing those fears directly, and perhaps having them quelled, game players throw up avoidance tactics. Sadly, they may not be aware that they are actually preventing themselves from having the benefits of a long term relationship while they bemoan the fact that they can't find the one special person they believe would make them happy.

Try this exercise if you want to identify a game you may be involved in:

Think of a situation you keep getting into, and which ends up with you feeling bad in some way. Then write down the answers to these questions, leaving 'mystery questions' until last.

1. *What is it that keeps happening to you?*
2. *How does it begin?*
3. *What happens then?*
4. ****mystery question****
5. *How does it continue?*
6. ****mystery question****
7. *How does it end?*
8. *How are you left feeling?*

*When you've answered these questions, go back to the ***mystery questions***. For question 4 ask 'What is it at this point you aren't saying, or avoiding asking for?'. For question 6 ask 'What is it that at this point you think the other person isn't saying?'*

*The whole set of answers will show you the pattern of the game. The ***mystery questions*** and answers will tell you what the game is all about, what's being avoided. Once you know that, you'll be able to choose whether to communicate those thoughts and feelings you've previously kept hidden rather than engage in an unproductive and repetitive game.*

If you get caught up in someone else's game then you have several options. You can, of course, continue to play — after all, some games are quite amusing as long as no-one is being hurt. If you don't want to go on playing, you can refuse point blank — 'I know that at this point I'd normally say . . . , but I don't want to get into that same old argument, so let's talk about something else.' Alternatively you could say 'I know that I usually get angry when you . . . but I'd like to tell you what I'm feeling now . . . '. You can always stop a game by giving an unexpected response.

Barrier Three

'Your better half'

The fear of losing yourself by losing your independence, is another barrier to good long term relationships. It's a fear of being swallowed up by the other person. In our culture this fear is often confirmed. Take, for example, women who automatically lose their own surnames when they marry, unless they opt otherwise. It can seem as if you stop being a whole person, and become half of one — you hear people introduce 'my better half'.

Anxiety about losing yourself is often unnecessary. Providing each person is willing to acknowledge their own and each other's needs, their individuality can be preserved. It's true that during the first phase of intimacy people often welcome and enjoy the feeling of being 'taken over' by the other. However, as the relationship develops each will rediscover their own sense of self and begin to separate. This comes as a surprise to some people who want to cling on to complete 'togetherness'.

No-one can take away your independence unless you give it to them. You may find yourself with someone who only feels secure by manipulating you into feeling dependent on them. They can seem to have power over you, because they give or deprive you of whatever it is you want from them. Claude Steiner, who helped develop Transactional Analysis (see pp. 78–80), wrote a book called *The Other Side of Power*, which shows how people who are insecure develop the ability to 'power play' others. 'All or nothing' is an example of the kind of strategies they use. The manipulator takes advantage of the fear someone may have of loss. It's a version of the childhood game 'If you don't play by my rules, I'll take my ball away'. Sulking is another example — where the sulker withdraws their affection or responsiveness in order to get what they want.

Others try to gain power by intimidation. Obviously big, loud-voiced people can intimidate others by their size or strength, but there are subtler methods too. People can be intimidated by interruptions, by having statistics or complicated facts quoted to them, by being forced to explain or defend themselves. Loss of independence is a real threat if you're teamed with a manipulator, but it isn't inevitable. What it's important to remember is the golden rule: you alone are responsible for what you do, think and feel. If you feel small, inadequate or swamped by someone, then at some level you are actually choosing to respond in that way. They may well be bigger, stronger and more devious than you, but you don't have to give over all your personal power to them.

If you find it difficult to stand up for yourself then there are ways of changing that, of increasing your confidence. Reading this book is a start, attending one of the many assertiveness courses would be another way, there are many ways to boost your own abilities. The thing to remember is that you cannot be taken over by anyone unless there is some way in which you are colluding with the situation.

Barrier Four

'Don't ever leave me'

Being left completely alone is one of the greatest terrors for human beings. The fear goes back to when, as babies, we realized we were actually separate from our mothers. That realization created a panic about who would care for us. Each time a baby wakes up and finds itself alone it cannot know someone is there until it has had enough experiences to provide it with the evidence. By then the awful fear that aloneness brings is implanted in our experience, and can be triggered off at different times in our adult life by the threat or event of someone close leaving us.

This fear is often responsible for people staying together when the relationship is dead, no intimacy or even any affection left. This, in some ways, is the reverse side of the coin to the fear of intimacy, and can be just as problematic. Many love songs and stories refer to the state of lovers 'being as one', and this is often how people feel in the first stages. However, as the relationship develops, and the partners need to move apart a bit, problems will arise if one or the other panics about possible separation. The fear of loneliness can impel someone to cover up their own needs in case they become too demanding and cause their partner to leave them.

Such fear makes direct and honest communication impossible. When a conflict arises such a person may make every effort to discount or deny the problem. The fear of separation can act as a kind of glue keeping people together, but it's like the old-fashioned glue which sticks things rigid and allows no room for flexible movement or freedom for the parties held together. Sometimes this 'stuck like glue' relationship is called the 'highest form of love' — people who are 'so close' they can't be separate for even a moment. It's unhealthy though, for when closely examined this kind of love keeps people imprisoned rather than helping them to develop or be free. In literature there are many examples of lovers who are so close they kill themselves or each other rather than be parted. Romeo and Juliet are probably the best-known examples — rather than be parted they commit suicide. This can be viewed as a noble act of love, or as an example of extreme passivity or dependence, resulting from the fear of separation.

What do you imagine if you think about a partner leaving you? Are you sad, angry, regretful, panic-stricken or terrified? Do you see yourself entirely alone and rejected by everyone? If someone really leaves you, then of course you will feel sad, angry, regretful, and you will need to mourn the loss, and live through a period of reassessment. If your feeling is one of overwhelming panic, or terror, maybe you need to explore what's really going on. If you could deal with the irrational part of your fear, the part that belongs to that frightened baby, you and your partner would be freer in the relationship.

The terror of being left can lead to extreme possessiveness and jealousy, almost a need to imprison the other person. If you try to do this you run the risk of overwhelming the other person to such an extent that they'll feel suffocated and need to break free, and you may lose them anyway. So if you can deal with your irrational fears, you can then relax and enjoy the present without needing to protect yourself from a fear-laden future.

Barrier Five

I know I can depend on you

If someone is afraid of being alone they may convince themselves that they have to depend on someone else. There are many couples who rely on each other's dependency and provide each other with support which they cannot give themselves. What this means is that if someone has difficulty satisfying their own needs they satisfy them by controlling their partner.

Imagine this scene:

> Alison has bought a new outfit. She is keen to get home from work so that she can show it to her boyfriend, Malcolm. She wonders during the day whether or not he'll like it. She rushes home and puts on the dress, and when Malcolm comes in and she's wearing it he doesn't comment. All through dinner Alison waits for the 'verdict'. If he doesn't like it she won't ever be happy wearing it. When the meal is finished, Malcolm smiles and says 'You look good'. Alison can relax. If he hadn't liked the dress she wouldn't have worn it again. Once her choice has got approval, it's acceptable, so she feels she is acceptable. Somehow she has given Malcolm so much power that he can decide whether or not she feels good about herself. A smile or a frown from him can change her perception of herself.

Many couples develop this kind of pattern, each depending on the other to tell them how to feel. It may seem from our little scene that Alison is the dependent partner, but in fact Malcolm depends on Alison whose passive response allows him to feel in charge. It's not unknown for people in power to surround themselves with 'yes' people, men and women who will approve of their every move. For the same reasons Malcolm needs his Alison, he depends on her depending on him.

Barrier Six

The great sacrifice

'I've given up all this for you' — the martyr role is very common in couples with a high (and likely to be unhealthy) degree of dependency. On the surface the person who plays the martyr seems a character over-brimming with goodness, making sacrifices so that the other can have just what they want. However it's also a very controlling role, inducing guilt and restricting the other person's freedom.

> Kevin was offered promotion by his company, which entailed moving to another town. His partner Bob's immediate reaction was of resistance to the move, since he had many friends and a job in their present hometown. Bob said nothing about his feelings, and so Kevin assumed that they would move house when he took up the promotion. They did move. Bob gave up his job and lost contact with his friends. Now, whenever Kevin wants something from Bob that he doesn't want to give, he often hears 'Haven't I done enough for you — I gave up everything for you'.

Self-imposed martyrdom like this seldom brings people closer together. In fact Kevin feels guilty and frustrated, and Bob resentful. The willingness to share is an important aspect of any good relationship, and there will be times when each person will be willing to forego their own desires if the other's need is greater, but not if the sacrifice will later be used as a weapon. Sharing can help you and your partner get closer, but you both have to be certain that you want to share.

Beware of rescuing. Rescuing is:

- doing something that you don't want to do.
- doing more than your share.
- doing something for which you're not asked.

It may seem that all these actions are merely displaying generosity and an understanding of the other person's needs. In reality, though, they can result in resentment being felt by the rescued and the rescuer. The problem is that every time you do something for someone you've actually deprived them of the opportunity to accept responsibility for themselves. In an emergency, or where the other person is too weak or young to take responsibility for themselves, then rescuing is necessary. After all, if you were walking down a river path and saw someone drowning you wouldn't stand on the bank wondering whether or not you should rescue them. You would be right in taking whatever action you could to save the drowning person. But if you're always 'good enough' to do someone's washing for them and 'rescue' them from this chore, they could feel you're manipulating them into being grateful, and you could feel resentful if they're unappreciative.

If you want to avoid being a rescuer, always check, when you're thinking of helping someone that:

- they want the help you're giving.
- you have a genuine wish to help them, and not be seen by them as good.
- you do not require them to be grateful.
- you don't require them to pay you back somehow.

Making these checks will ensure that you don't get involved in underhanded dependency games.

Barrier Seven

Old habits die hard

Many of the barriers we've identified are the result of patterns of behaviour established in childhood which seem to recur over and over again. The fact that they don't produce satisfying results doesn't seem to stop them repeating. Claude Steiner, in his book *Scripts People Live*, describes how in everyday life people seem to repeat their main life-script in miniature. For instance, the response of someone to a household crisis, like the washing machine overflowing, will reflect their response to other life crises.

(a) They may blame the washing machine — 'That's the trouble with machines, you just can't trust them.'
(b) They may blame themselves — 'If I hadn't put so much washing in . . . it's all my fault.'
(c) They may see it as fate — 'I knew things were going too well, something had to go wrong.'
(d) They may see it as yet another example of how much a victim of life they are — 'This kind of thing always happens to me.'
(e) They may see it as a problem to be solved — 'Now, what can I do to fix this?'

You can probably think of lots more reactions. The likelihood is that whatever the reaction, it will reflect that person's perception of how their life runs.

Try this exercise to identify some aspects of your 'script':

Think of a recent event when you were involved in some kind of problem — not necessarily a major crisis, but something which at the time provoked an emotional response from you.

What thoughts went through your head at the time — about you, about other people involved, about the world in general?

Were any of these thoughts familiar ones?

What emotional response did you have?

Were these feelings familiar?

What did you actually do?

Was this a usual response?

The patterns which make up our script are created from many influences. Take, for instance, your place in the family. Whether you were an only child, a first-born with brothers and sisters, a middle child, or the youngest, will have great influence on how you see life when you are a very small child.

As an only child, you would have responded mainly to the needs and wishes of adults, so in later life you may find it easier to make lasting relationships with people who are older, or in an authority role with you, or conversely with people who are younger or with whom you are in some authority role. As a child you may not have had a great deal of experience of your peers, of living with brothers and sisters around the same age, so you may not have developed the necessary skills to survive in the hurly-burly of life with people who have an equal position to you.

Another problem for the only child is that since adults can usually do things much better than children, they are constantly having to match themselves against those standards. So they may learn never to be satisfied unless they can achieve more than those around them. Conversely they may be so praised by their proud parents for small achievements that they get an over-inflated idea of how good they are and feel everyone should praise them.

A first-born child has to learn to contend with competition, since when the second baby is born the first no longer has the undivided attention of its parents. Whereas the second-born often experiences fewer demands, and less pressure to excel, they may suffer the problem of constantly trying to catch up with and be just as good as their brothers or sisters.

The last-born, the baby of the family, has to cope with the feeling that everyone else is bigger and more powerful. They may well develop skills in getting what they want by manipulating others, since they cannot compete on equal grounds.

These are just a few suggestions about how one aspect of our early development – birth order – can influence our whole perception of our place in the world, and so, inevitably, our ability to relate with others.

If you'd like to consider how your place in your family may still be influencing you, try this:

When you have some time to yourself, without being interrupted, close your eyes and imagine yourself back in your childhood, sitting at the table having a meal with the family. Notice who talks to who. Do you have difficulty getting a word in edgeways? Is there someone definitely 'in charge'? Are you allowed to say what you think? Or do you have to be careful not to upset someone? Are you able to get as much as you want to eat, or do you have to fight for your share, or are you told off for leaving food on the plate? Is there someone who gets favourable treatment from the adults?

When you've imagined the scene, and remembered as much as you can about what it used to be like, ask yourself those questions in relation to how life is for you now.

For instance, do you still feel that you have to fight for your share? Or that you can't say no if someone asks you if you want something to eat? Do you still go quiet in a group? Is there still a 'parent' watching how you behave?

Such scripts can be understood, and overcome. Once you begin to understand your own habitual way of seeing and responding to the world, you can begin to change your way of behaving, if you want to. You may have been the youngest and weakest in the family once upon a time, but not necessarily now, and so your habitual response may be completely inappropriate and even damaging. You can, if you wish, put aside those aspects of your script that create barriers to good relationships, and learn new ways of being with people.

Barrier Eight

A starring role — or a bit part?

Our lives can be seen like a film in which we play a part. The role we play is determined by many factors of which our inner script is one. Another is our culture. If you're female, there will be certain expectations as to how you should behave, just as there are expectations on men. Society has guidelines on what makes an acceptable husband or wife, a good mother or child, and so on. All those outside factors will be nudging in, trying to take over your script and encourage you to play the part the way they visualize the character. Remember, it's your own movie, and if you want to have a starring role in it, you need to write your own script. You may wish to seek guidance from other people, but if you let them write it all you'll end up merely playing a bit part in your own production.

Breaching the barriers

When you think about all the problems which can stand in the way of long-term relationships, it's easy to get the impression that it's all hopeless and that you must rely on pure luck to meet the kind of person you can relate to easily. This isn't really the case.

The advantage of identifying barriers which may block you is that as your understanding grows you'll be better able to shift the blocks.

So if things aren't going the way you want, the first thing to do is analyse what's actually happening.

Here are a series of questions which may help you do that:

1. *What is actually happening now?*
2. *What isn't happening?*
3. *How does it affect you?*
4. *How does it affect the other person/people?*
5. *What would you prefer to be happening?*
6. *What would you have to do to ensure success?*
7. *What are you willing to do?*
8. *How is that different from what you're already doing?*
9. *What stands in the way of your changing?*
10. *What is the worst that could happen?*
11. *How would you deal with that?*
12. *How might you sabotage yourself?*
13. *Is there some way in which others could help you?*
14. *What are others' expectations of you?*

The answers to these questions will help you analyse what is really happening, and what you might do about it.

The exercises earlier in this chapter will have helped you identify aspects of your script which will still be influencing you, so you need to consider whether there is anything which would benefit from thinking about and working on.

If you have identified a problem which has several elements the next stage is to decide which aspect of the problem you want to deal with first. You can only work on one thing at a time, and as you succeed in changing that, you'll be able to move on to other aspects of the problem. Set yourself small goals, and if you're working together with your partner, set them together. If you see something as an overwhelming problem, with so many things needing doing it all seems impossible, you'll never get anywhere because it will all seem too much. Breaking things down into small goals means each achievement will lead you towards the main changes you want to make.

Do remember that the goals you set yourself and each other should be realistic, measurable, specific, adequate, and within your control — it's no good trying to change the weather!

Making it work

At the beginning of this chapter we said that we couldn't provide a blueprint of a good relationship, since individuals have so many different needs. Having concentrated so far on potential problem areas it may seem as if it's all gloom, doom and difficulty. That's not quite the case though. You may not already have a clear idea in your mind of what a good relationship would look like to you. If not then the following pointers may help you. With your aims in mind you will find it a lot easier to pinpoint problems as and when they arise.

Good relationships aren't only those you may wish to have with sexual partners — friendships, family, parenting and even working relationships may benefit from these guidelines.

Find common ground If you've got nothing in common, no shared values or interests then relating will be difficult. You don't have to agree with each other all the time, but you do need to have some understanding of the other's view of the world. You need to have some meeting points, so that when you talk to each other there are certain things which you can take for granted as being understood. This common ground might include how decisions will be taken, a commitment to agreements being kept, an understanding of how much time you'll spend together or apart, how money will be spent, and so on. If there are no agreements of this kind then the relationship will feel insecure.

Fix the problem, not the person It's impossible to have a problem-free life. In a relationship it can be tempting always to see a problem as someone else's fault, so a lot of energy may go into trying to change them. It's not possible for one person to change another — the best you can hope to do is offer the other person an opportunity to change, perhaps by altering your own behaviour, or by asking them directly for what you want. The other person will only change if doing so will have advantages for them. In an alive and healthy relationship the partners will work together to solve problems rather than waste energy by trying to change each other.

Have fun Children seek out friends they can play with, and the most enjoyable childhood memories are likely to be of times when you were with someone you liked, who liked you, and with whom you could share fun and games. It's no different for adults. There is a child in us all, and that child needs to have the chance to express itself. So, another sign of a good relationship is the ability and willingness to 'let your hair down' with each other, maybe playing games, or going dancing or walking, or enjoying making love together, or just being together. We all need fun in our lives, especially in what may otherwise seem the serious business of relationships.

Look after each other There will be times when one or other person in the relationship is feeling hurt, depressed, lonely, frightened, or perhaps ill. Though over-dependency on each other can be a barrier, a good relationship does need each to have a willingness to look after the other when they are feeling weak or needy.

Work it out It can help if you work out between you how you both want the relationship to operate. Some couples have gone so far as to draw up contracts about who is responsible for what, and marriage itself involves a contract with it. If it helps to sort out who'll phone who, who'll do what bits of cleaning, who'll look after finances and so on, then do so. Without this it's easy to fall into the trap of believing that your partner agrees with your way of handling things when they don't at all. Don't assume that how you've done things in the past is the 'right' way — you may need to negotiate.

Face complications A relationship isn't static, nor is it an island, and outside pressures will take their toll. One or both partners' careers may impinge, unemployment can rock the boat, the arrival of a child may shift the balance, family problems may pull one partner away for a while. If your general communication is good then you'll probably face and deal with such changes and complications, if not then you may wonder why your 'perfect' world has suddenly gone wrong.

Complications can be created in many different ways. The happy days of 'coupledom' can lose their shine when family or friends try to influence the course of a relationship, even try to split it up. But there are few complications larger than the birth of a baby, even if greeted with delight by both parents, it will create changes. Babies don't instantly fit in with their family's wishes. They wake up when they're hungry and demand to be fed — whatever the time. The fact that most adults organize their lifestyle around being awake for sixteen hours and then asleep for eight is news to a baby. So the parents get very tired. Exhaustion creates stress which can make people snap.

It's an extraordinary fact that, although most people become parents, very few of them have any real education in how to *be* a parent. Most learning is done 'on the job'. This means that the parent may be not only fatigued, but also anxious about doing the right thing. Should they feed the baby when it cries, or should they create some disciplined structure? Should they leave a baby out in the air, or should they keep it in a warm room? Should they call a doctor if the baby has spots? The questions are endless and for most of them there are no right answers, only opinions. So the next anxiety is which 'expert opinion' to follow, since you can be sure of finding several different ideas to choose from.

So the couple who only had each other to consider before the arrival of the baby, now have a third person — and one who is a hard taskmaster — to take into account. It isn't difficult to see how this could affect a relationship. Fatigue and anxiety shorten tempers, relaxed sex may become an enjoyment of the past, money may become short; spontaneous recreation is no longer possible, disagreements over childcare may arise — the list goes on.

The complications can increase as the children grow up. Reaching agreements as to how the children are to be brought up, how they are to be educated, dealing with feelings of competition, are all issues which may have to be addressed.

Another kind of complication arises when one partner's career development means a drastic change in lifestyle. For instance, someone who is extremely successful in business may begin moving in very different circles, or one partner may get an offer of a job in a different part of the country. Changes like these will of course affect both people in the relationship. Redundancy can also create problems. No-one expects to become redundant when they start out in a job, and so very few are prepared either financially or emotionally for the event if it occurs.

Sometimes people realize quite late in a career that they would really like to be doing something else. If they do change, that may mean financial restrictions and perhaps increased tension if risks are involved. If they don't change, they may feel increasingly dissatisfied with life as a whole.

Money, particularly the lack of it, can cause complications. Love, of course, is free. Living is not. It is a naive and romantic view that money is unnecessary for a happy and contented life. This view is usually put forward by people who actually have enough.

These are just some examples of how complications can arise

through external pressures on a relationship. Some of these will be resolved through good communication and a willingness to face the problems; some of them cannot be resolved and so decisions will have to be made regarding actions according to the wishes and needs of each person. Not every situation of this kind has a happy ending. It may be that people will decide to split up because they cannot come to any amicable arrangement.

Being on your own

Though we've spent a great deal of time talking about healthy partnerships and the anxiety caused by real or threatened separation, being on your own has its advantages too. Being solo, whether by choice or circumstance, is valuable in developing your own autonomy, your independence, and surprisingly it can be good for developing a present or future relationship. If you can stand on your own feet you won't need to tread on anyone else's.

Many loving couples go through periods of separation and find that their relationship is stronger as a result. Being on your own provides an opportunity to develop a whole set of skills which are necessary for independence, for making you a 'whole' person. Being alone is not failure or disaster, but there may be particular skills you need to learn.

Coping with your feelings

Finding yourself alone can lead to anger, depression, jealousy, anxiety, loneliness and/or panic. In order to get on with your life you will have to face these feelings and come to terms with them.

Some people, if left by a lover, will become intensely jealous and obsessed with staying in contact. They may track the person down and follow or harass them with phone calls or letters. Others create a whirlwind lifestyle, entering into many casual relationships or building a social life in which there's no time to breathe, in an attempt to wipe out all memory of their ex-partner. Whilst these reactions may be understandable, they don't help the individual to move through the experience and learn from it.

It would be wiser to accept the painful feelings, face them and try to deal with them, and learn from them rather than try to escape from them. Escape isn't possible anyway, only temporary avoidance. There is a recognized grief process of bereavement which doesn't only happen when someone dies. Separation, divorce, and other losses follows a similar pattern. It's almost as if we need to go through the anger and pain to finish off one scene before we can gainfully enter another.

There are techniques for dealing with loss; one is to pretend you are an observer. When thoughts and feelings connected with your loss arise, make a detailed analysis of them. How long do the feelings last? What physical reaction do you experience? What are you actually thinking?

None of this will change what has happened. Nothing will ever change the past. What it will do is allow you to become more aware of your emotions and better prepared to cope when it happens again. Notice, too, that even painful emotions don't last forever. If you time how long you feel depressed, anxious, jealous and so on, you'll notice that the intensity of your feelings diminishes and disappears for a while before reappearing. As time goes on the gaps between those painful emotions gets longer. You're recovering from your loss.

Expand yourself No, we don't mean put on weight or build up muscle. If you've been involved in a close, almost exclusive relationship, then separation can be devastating. It can seem that your whole world has fallen apart. Not only do you no longer have the companionship of the other, but you're left with nothing to do but focus on your own thoughts and feelings about your loss. In fact, being alone can provide great opportunities for renewing or developing interests.

Getting out your paints or guitar, starting a new evening class or joining a social club, won't bring back the person or put together a broken love affair. What new activities can do, however, is help you improve the relationship you have with yourself, boost your self-confidence and ability to cope in the world. After all, if you're going to have to live with yourself for a while, you are likely to enjoy it more if you discover that you are an interesting, active person.

Nobody can tell you what activities will suit you best — you have to decide that for yourself. Shifting off your backside and doing something, though, will help, because the more you take responsibility for yourself and your own enjoyment, the more easily you will recover from the distress of separation. Sitting around blaming your unhappiness on the other person effectively paralyses you — they may have had a hand in the past, but now you need to look at the present and future, and that's in your hands. It's as well to remember that people who are happy with their own company and who lead lives they find interesting are a more tempting and attractive prospect for other people.

5

Body Works

So far we've concentrated on what goes on in our minds. In this chapter attention is paid to our bodies. After all, we experience everything that happens to us through our bodies, and just as understanding our minds helps us change and develop in the way we want, so understanding our bodies ensures we get as much pleasure as possible from loving relationships.

To start at the beginning: men and women are physically different from the moment of conception. A girl begins from two X chromosomes, a boy has one X and one Y. Of course you can't see chromosomes, but the physical differences these produce give young children hours of entertaining curiosity playing the game of 'why have you got different parts from me?'

In baby and childhood explorations many discover that rubbing their genitals gives them a pleasurable sensation, but whilst adults looking on may be shocked at such early 'sexual' awareness, this isn't sexual in the way adults know it. It's yet another exciting discovery the child is making, no different from the fascination of watching their own feet move, or the pleasure and comfort from sucking a thumb, or the curiosity about their bodily functions.

Real sexual awakenings happen at puberty when the body's complex hormone system brings a few more hormones into play, producing physical and emotional changes.

Child to teenager

As children both sexes are free of pubic and underarm hair and have scant body hair. Neither little boys nor girls sweat as much as adults. It's not until about 12 or 13 that girls's 'apocrine' or adult sweat glands develop, with boys it's a little later, about 13 to 15. This is why young teenagers may suddenly get lectures on personal hygiene and be presented with bottles of underarm deodorant — they hadn't needed them before.

Just prior to the perspiration boom is the growth spurt — another expensive bit for parents! Girls of around 10 or 11 and boys of around 12 or 13 may seem to grow almost overnight. The growth isn't all visible — the heart, for instance, nearly doubles in size. The lungs grow and the blood pressure is altered. Of course how tall a person becomes depends on what they've inherited from their parents — short parents tend to produce short offspring, but other factors such as nutrition are important. If you look back at our ancestors, who had tougher lives and poorer diets, we're mostly giants by comparison. The adolescent growth spurt carries on until about 16 for girls and 18 for boys.

Girls are born with their complete reproductive system. The ovaries, though immature, already contain enough ova (eggs) to last the woman a lifetime. Adjoining the ovaries, which lie on either side of the body near the hip bones, are the fallopian tubes which lead into the uterus (womb), which in turn joins with the vagina. The connecting entrance from the vagina to the womb is called the cervix and can be felt as a nobbly bit, rather like the end of a nose, at the top of the vagina. All that is internal. On the woman's external genital area, in front of the opening to the vagina, is her clitoris, a small hooded lump which can be allied, in sensitivity, to the male penis. A female also has genital 'lips' called the labia majora and the labia minora. Sometimes the inner lips, the labia minora which are wrinkled and fleshy, hang lower than the outer, fuller labia majora. This, or small, hidden labia, are both normal.

One of the most obvious changes a girl notices at puberty is the start of menstruation. For boys it will be the growth of their penis. In both cases the body has begun preparing for these changes several years in advance. A part of the brain called the hypothalmus starts to send messages to the pituitary gland, at the base of the brain, and in turn the pituitary releases hormones. The first is the growth hormone. Then, for both sexes, comes the Follicle Stimulating Hormone (usually called, for simplicity, FSH).

In girls FSH tells the ovaries it's time to start ripening the ova (eggs) but first, the follicles they rest in must grow. Once the follicles are stimulated they in turn produce oestrogen, a hormone which will play a regular part in the menstrual cycle, but is also responsible for aiding the growth of breasts and genitals. Girls at this stage of development will also start to put on more body fat, predominantly over the hips, thighs, breasts and upper arms — they begin to get more 'shapely'. One breast may begin developing before the other, and it's quite normal, anyway, for adult women to have one breast a little larger than the other.

As the levels of oestrogen increase, the hypothalmus gets a message back to slow up on the FSH it's been nudging the pituitary to release. Then the pituitary releases luteinizing hormone (LH), which tells the follicles in the ovaries it's time to burst one so that an ovum (egg) can be released. An ovum is released, on average, once every 28 days. The collapsed follicle it leaves behind (called the corpus luteum) carries on releasing oestrogen, but adds to that another hormone called progesterone. The purpose of progesterone is to prepare the lining of the womb to accept a fertilized egg. If the ovum isn't fertilized then the levels of both oestrogen and progesterone fall, causing the womb lining to be shed and leave the body. This bleeding we know as periods.

A girl's first period usually happens between the ages of 11 and 14. She may get a good indication of when to expect it by asking her mother when she started, as mothers and daughters tend to have similar menstrual patterns, especially the start (the menarche) and finish (the menopause). Before the first period a girl is likely to notice a whitish discharge from the vagina. Once a regular menstrual cycle is established she can, with careful monitoring, know which part of the cycle she is in by her discharge. At ovulation it gets thicker, more the consistency of egg white. Generally a period occurs about two weeks after an egg has been released from the ovary.

Initially periods may be quite irregular, but they should steadily settle into a pattern. Women will often need to know the date of their periods, so it's best to keep a check in a diary.

The hormones FSH and LH affect the male body too. Here they work on the testicles (balls). Once activated, the testes produce the male hormone, testosterone. Under the influence of testosterone the testicles begin to grow and the skin around them, the scrotum, darkens. This starts at about 11 or 12. Following on, the penis first lengthens, then broadens. About a year after this growth begins the boy may experience his first wet dream, when he gets an erection in the night and ejaculates semen. This can be as much of a shock for boys as the first period is for girls if they're not prepared for it.

Average penis length is 3½″ (9 cm) from base to tip when flaccid. This is average, remember, and though many men worry about their size there's very rarely need to. When erect the size can change quite dramatically, so comparing in gents' showers is a bit of a wasted exercise, especially as then the male will be looking at the whole of others' and down on his own so not seeing its full length!

During their teens boys change shape too. Their shoulders

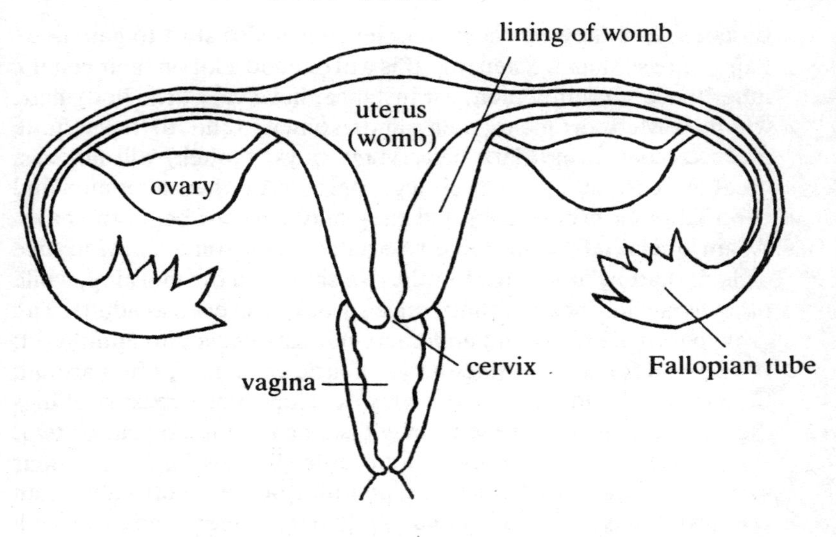

Internal

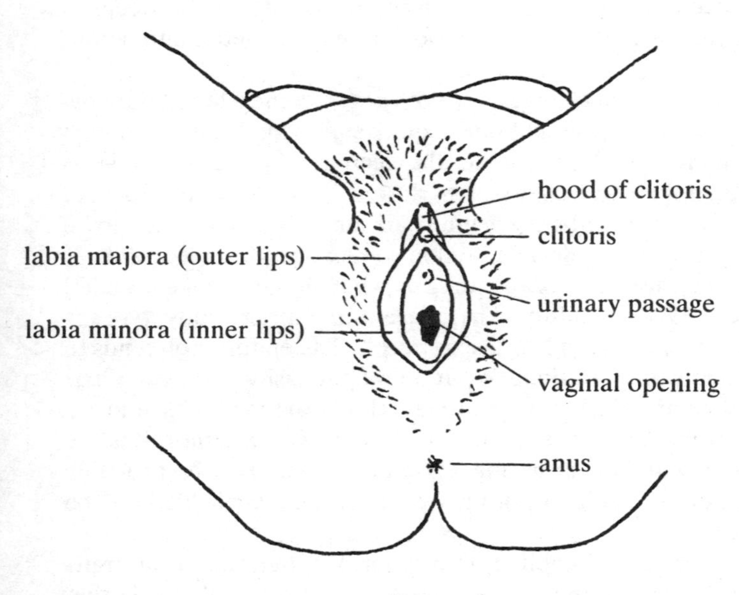

External

The Female Reproductive System

broaden, and they get more muscley. They also start to gain body hair, more so than women, but this will depend a lot on their genetic inheritance. Oriental men, for instance, have very little body hair, whereas Mediterranean men, and women, tend to have quite profuse, coarse and dark hair. Many boys, though, will notice a great increase in hair on their legs, perhaps on their abdomen and chest (though not always) and they may need to begin to shave. Again, facial hair is extremely variable, with some showing 'five o'clock shadow' not long after they've shaved in the morning, while others may only need to shave once a week or so even as adults. The growth of male chest and abdomen hair carries on into adulthood. It's normal for some women to get a little chest hair, often around the nipples. Incidentally, boys may develop small breast swellings during adolescence. These usually disappear within a year or two.

One of the outwardly most noticeable changes for boys is their voice breaking. Girls' voices deepen too, but less noticeably than boys, who may sound deep and manly one moment and produce a high squeak the next. To facilitate this deepening voice the larynx, or voicebox, begins to grow at about 13 or 14, and this may mean the appearance of an 'adam's apple' in the throat. The voice deepens about a year after this growth, though it may not settle until about 16 or 17.

All these physical changes, for both sexes, come a lot earlier now than once was the case. No-one is quite sure why this is so, though it's often assumed it's due to the increase in living standards compared to our ancestors. It's slowed down though, from an advance of four months every ten years, and it's now thought to be about a month every decade, and in some places has stood still.

The timing also varies depending on what physical shape the child will end up as an adult. There are three basic body types – endomorph, mesomorph and ectomorph. The endomorph tends to be the cuddly type, inclined to put on weight easily, have curly hair and small teeth. Mesomorphs are muscley with long limbs, and are inclined to have large teeth and thick hair. The ectomorph is the lanky type, with long arms and legs and a thin body, who probably finds it quite difficult to put on weight. Their hair is likely to be straight.

Most of us are a combination of 'morphs', but one of the traits may overide the others. How your 'type' affects puberty is that endomorphs and mesomorphs tend to hit puberty earlier than ectomorphs. This may have something to do with body weight, as certainly girls aren't likely to have their first period until they've reached at least 7 stone in weight. In fact in later years, after puberty, if a girl's weight drops significantly this may halt her periods.

Once it's working

These dramatic changes of puberty should come to a halt at about 17 or 18. That's not the end of the story though, more of a beginning. As already mentioned, a girl's periods may be irregular to start with. There are other facts it's worth knowing. Accepting that periods are natural and necessary is a good start. If a girl has been led to believe that they are a 'curse' or 'woman's suffering' then chances are she will suffer. One line of thought is that many of the period pains women endure are caused by the girl, or woman, dreading the event, and sub-consciously clenching the muscles in the uterus. This makes the necessary work of evacuating the uterine lining more difficult, and hence painful. It's true that those taught to welcome periods as a sign of maturing seem to have less bother, but let's look, anyway, at how to deal with difficulties which may otherwise blight a woman every month.

Day One in the menstrual cycle is the first day of bleeding. For some this is virtually uneventful — no pain, no problems, just a sign that all is in working order. Others may get backache and pain in the lower abdomen. Although retiring to bed with a hot water bottle and a couple of painkillers may ease the pain, and may occasionally be what's called for, it's a pity if about twelve times a year a woman has to become an invalid due to a perfectly natural event. She may not feel like it at the time, but often exercise, swimming, dancing, or even a brisk walk can cure the pain just as quickly.

Yoga can be particularly good for this cramping pain. To benefit this way from yoga you really need to practice the techniques often, to get the muscles into good and stretchy tone. Yoga classes are now commonplace and any teacher will guide you on exercises particularly good for the pelvic region. Encouraging the muscles to work and do their job effectively may solve pain problems, or at least ease them which may be enough.

The bleeding itself may last from two to eight days and the amount is probably far less than many women think. Over the whole time it's likely to only be between half and a full cup's worth, and the blood is mixed with dead cells and mucus. The flow itself may vary over the days with the first few days often being the heaviest. What kind of sanitary protection to wear is a matter of individual choice, but there's no reason why young girls shouldn't use tampons from the beginning if they wish.

There are a lot of myths surrounding menstruation. Some cultures say a woman is 'unclean' during this time, but there's no reason why that should be. Certainly the old wives' tale that a woman shouldn't wash her hair during a period is utter nonsense, but ignorance breeds many peculiar 'wisdoms'. As long as towels or tampons are changed several times a day there's nothing unclean about it. Quite the reverse really, as a period could be seen as a cleansing operation, clearing the womb to prepare for the coming cycle.

During a period a woman may find that various other parts of her body are affected. It's common, for instance, for constipation to occur a few days prior to Day One. If she's severely bunged up this in itself could cause period pain, but a mild change in pattern may be worth nothing more than noting. She may also feel a little bloated during the days beforehand and notice, towards the end of bleeding that she's visiting the loo more often – the water her body has stored is passing. Her skin may be sensitive to the hormone changes and produce a few spots. These too will usually pass.

When the bleeding is over the woman moves towards ovulation. For most this goes by unnoticed, but a few women feel a bit of pain in the lower abdomen at their mid-cycle and perhaps come to realize this is the follicle releasing the egg. However, it's easily confused with the pain from wind in the gut! Though it's rare, it's also possible to bleed a little at ovulation. Both phenomena are referred to as mittelschmerz (middle pain) by the medical profession.

The next phase is the worst for those unfortunate women who suffer from the problems known as pre-menstrual tension (PMT) or the pre-menstrual syndrome (PMS). Sufferers complain that they feel bloated, irritable, depressed, even to the point of feeling suicidal. For many this is simply rectified by ensuring good nutrition, rest, exercise and fresh air — basically taking care of themselves. Skipping breakfast or going on a starvation diet, for example, are likely to cause problems during this time when many women find they crave sugary foods and probably do need energy-giving sustenance to help their bodies along.

Studies on supplementing vitamin intake, particularly vitamin B6, have shown some positive responses, but it's important to keep balance, as too much of anything, even a vitamin, can be as bad as too little. Specific advice on dietary suggestions for dealing with pre-menstrual problems can be obtained from the Pre-Menstrual Tension Advisory Service (address on page 159). Another line of thought is that hormone help, in particular progesterone, can solve the problem. A doctor's prescription is necessary for this, or other drug help.

Some women notice a boost in their libido (sex drive) around ovulation, and for others this may occur just before menstruation. How much of this is a psychological desire to conceive, or not, is unknown, but it's one factor to consider, along with hormone changes. Certainly for women who are trying to conceive the start of a period may be depressing for obvious reasons.

Now, to move up the body to the other female attributes — breasts. These too can be a cause of great anxiety to some who feel they're too small, too big, or 'different' in some way. As women don't get that many chances of comparing themselves, except perhaps to 'Page Three' specially selected specimens, it's easy to overlook the fact that every pair of breasts is different, just as our faces are different. It's also true that human nature being what it is, we inevitably hanker after what we haven't got. Just as we can wish for straight hair if ours is curly, or vice versa, so it can be with boobs, except you can't have them adjusted as easily to suit fashion.

Fashion generates a lot of anxiety, and there are trends in what's 'desirable' bust size of the moment. Twiggy set a trend for small-breasted women, whereas previously stars like Marilyn Monroe had sported sizeable attributes. Our bodies aren't like clothes which can be tailored to suit the moment. By and large, we have to make do and accept what nature, diet and exercise have produced, unless you decide to go in for expensive (and not always successful) cosmetic surgery. Remember, though, that just as breast size varies so do the tastes of those who find women sexually desirable and there is more, anyway, to femininity, sexuality — call it what you will — than a pair of mammary glands.

Normal, healthy breasts are made up of fibrous tissue, fat, and ducts for delivering milk to the nipple for breast-feeding, when called for. There is no muscle in the breast, though behind it the pectoral muscles aid support, so exercise can't actually change the shape of the breasts, though toning up the muscles behind may make some difference. Gaining or losing weight may alter the breast shape and size. Pregnancy may leave tell-tale signs, and the contraceptive pill can prompt breast increase in some women, though often to those who don't want it. Other than these factors (or surgery) there's not much you can do which will have any significant effect, so it's as well to accept what nature has given you. Good bras are valuable for some, especially heavy-breasted women who may be uncomfortable without, and sufferers from mastitis (painful lumpy breasts) are likely to be more comfortable wearing a supportive bra both day and night. Many, though, don't need bras for comfort, but may choose to wear them for cosmetic purposes.

Just as the breast itself comes in umpteen varieties, so do nipples, both in size and colouring. It's perfectly normal to have one or both nipples inverted (not pointing outwards), unless this suddenly happens whereas previously they'd been proud (more of that in the chapter on Sexual Health). It's also normal to have a few hairs around the nipple, but if a woman wishes to remove them she should trim them, not pluck out in this sensitive area.

While we're on women, just one last word (or two) and that's on body hair. Though many women get anxious about it, the fact is that pubic hair was around long before bikinis and so it may not be neatly hidden. The fashion in our society is for women to seem as hair-free as possible. There's fine hair all over the body, but on women their legs, under-arms and pubic hair will be darker and coarser and this body hair sometimes causes unnecessary worry. Body hair can be bleached, or removed by using depilatory creams, shaving (inadvisable, as it can cause increased growth, but some people do it), or waxing, or it can be killed off by electrolysis. For cosmetic and fashion reasons some women may wish to do this, but female body hair itself is not abnormal nor any cause for alarm or concern. Some darker hair on the face is also normal, though profuse growth may signal a hormone imbalance and might be worth checking with a doctor. This is rarely the case though.

Men too

Over to the men, whose system is almost as complex. Few men get real education about how their reproductive system works. They'll know about erections, but whereas women, because of contraceptive needs and pregnancy, are likely to come across the medical terms and workings of their body, men don't often have the need to talk about or know their internal workings. So what goes on?

Sperm production is going on all the time. The average male will make about 200 million sperm daily. They are made in the testes (another word for testicles) and stored in an organ called the

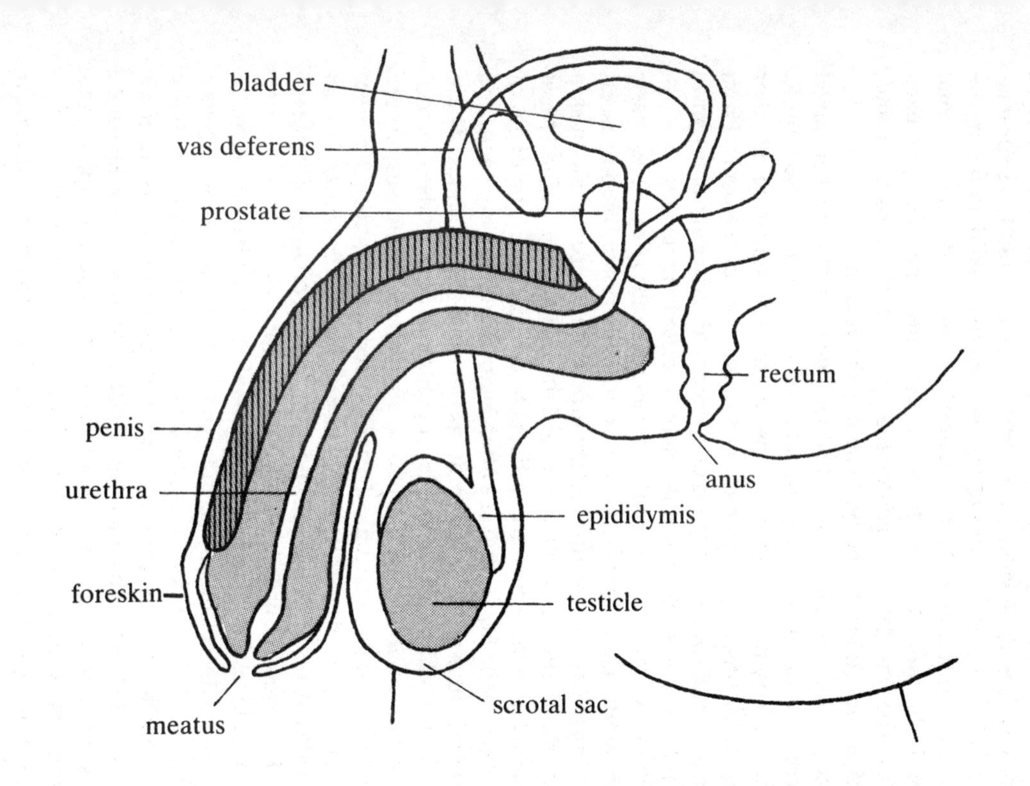

The Male Reproductive System

epididymis (plural epididymides). The testes and epididymides lie alongside each other in the scrotal sacs, the two sacs being referred to as the scrotum. Incidentally, the left testicle is often the larger of the two. Sperm are about 1/500th of an inch long and take 60 to 72 days to mature. Before maturation they are referred to as spermatocytes. There's over a foot to travel from the epididymides to the tip of the penis and when this action is summoned, due to sexual arousal, the route is through the vas deferens (one tube from each testis). The vas deferens guides the sperm to the prostate gland, which is tucked inside the body nearer the rectum.

The prostate produces fluid called seminal fluid which, when mixed with the sperm, make up semen, which is white and relatively thick. From the prostate the semen travels into the urethra which, at other times, is the tube through which urine passes out of the penis. From there it's a well-known story, except perhaps it's not commonly known that the opening in the tip of the penis is called the meatus.

Penises come in a variety of shapes and sizes. The basic components inside the loose skin are spongy tissue, blood vessels and the urethra. At the tip, in its natural state, there's a fold of skin called the foreskin. Rolled forward it resembles a hood. Most differences of the penis are noticeable on erection. The angle of erection may be horizontal or vertical with degrees in between, and a man may himself have different 'angles' at different times. There may be a bend inwards of the erect penis and bends sideways too, none of which are likely to cause any problems. However, severe changes in erectile state are best reported to a doctor. An erect penis is often significantly larger than its former flaccid self — on average the excited organ will be 5–7 in (13–18 cm) long, with larger flaccid penises often showing least expansion.

It's not necessary to tell any male about the sensitivity of the male genitalia. A direct hit to the area can immobilize the owner with severe pain. The reason such sensitive parts are outside the body rather than held inside bony protection is temperature. Sperm don't like to be too hot or too cold. This is why on a winter's day the whole system shrinks towards the body, while in a hot atmosphere the scrotum will drop to let the testes hang lower.

Sometimes one testicle retreats inside the body. If it comes down at times, and by the end of puberty stays descended, then all is well. If it remains undescended, however, a doctor should be consulted in case surgery is needed to protect future health. One testicle, incidentally, is enough to father children.

Because this entire area is sensitive it's advisable for men to wear support (jock straps) for sports. These hold the penis and scrotum up against the body, so at less risk of accidental injury. For sports like cricket, more robust protection is used.

So who is this person?

Whilst the body changes, the psyche too is growing, figuring out how to relate to the rest of the world. It's gaining experience and learning how to get what it wants without being hurt too much. The fact is that we often grow through painful experiences, and growing up is painful.

Adapting to very obvious physical changes can be difficult. Most teenagers spend a lot of time examing themselves in the mirror, checking growth, checking spots, adjusting their hair. They start to become in charge of their own body, wash their own hair, are allowed to lock the bathroom door. If the mind has difficulty adjusting to these physical changes it may pick on one part of the body and make a scapegoat of it.

We're often encouraged to make our bodies take blame or credit for our social success. If your hair looks right admirers will flock — at least, so the advertisers tell us. Some companies stand a lot to gain by encouraging the belief that if you're too fat then everyone else will be disgusted by you. So if you don't make a social hit whenever you want to, you may turn to a diet for a solution, when in reality it's your own behaviour, or someone else's, which may be the true problem.

Some people try to hide behind their bodies too — use them as defensive barriers. Subconsciously it may be felt that a wall of fat will keep others away, which protects you from confronting a possible problem directly. If this is the case then any attempts at dieting will fail anyway, because the true reasons for a problem haven't been tackled. Similarly anorexics who try to disappear into a skeletal frame may imprison themselves by a diet and strict physical regime and still feel they're failing, because the central problem, their emotional life, isn't receiving the attention it needs. Trying to get control of our lives is a desirable adolescent and adult goal, but if that control becomes difficult for some reason, we can try to impose control elsewhere, and blame that for the problem. 'Elsewhere' could be weight, height, colouring, gender, race, sexual preferences, the nose, the breasts, the penis, the eyes, the teeth.

Though physical differences may seem a catastrophe as a teenager, when everyone is trying to look like their mates or model themselves on ideals, it's as well to remember that what's beautiful to one person may be unattractive to another. And just as no personality is perfect so no body is either. There may well be room for improvement — how you stand and carry yourself, for example, is an important part of body language. But you don't need the perfect body (whatever that may be) to use body language. We all do it. Present yourself with openness and acceptance of yourself and others are more likely to find you attractive.

Reject your body and you reject yourself. Just as it's important to like yourself and be kind to yourself, so it's important to get to know your body and accept it. Of course you should do what you can to help it. Bodies like, and respond well to, exercise, good nutrition, fresh air, rest and so on. But work with what you've got, not what you envy someone else for.

Exploring your body is an important part of acceptance. If you don't know what's there, what it feels like to touch, and to look at, then it's easy to get frightened through ignorance, frightened of what you think may be there than what actually is. So, if necessary use a mirror and look in your mouth, at your back, under your arms, examine your feet and legs, look at your chest and examine your genitals. Self-examination isn't only necessary for acceptance, but as a part of health. If you know what you look like when you're healthy, then you'll have a better idea of whether your body is ill.

Accepting your own body, feeling good in it, and being good to it, will help in attracting other people. People often get anxious that if they don't possess what they consider to be the perfect body that they'll stand less chance, or no chance, of attracting others. Leaving aside the fact their own judgement may be overly critical, attraction between two people is based on far more than shape. For a kick-off it seems we humans tend to be physically attracted to people who look fairly similar to ourselves, if not by facial looks then by style. Similar taste in dress can suggest that you might share views — it's not very likely, for instance, that someone with an outrageous pink hair-style would rush for a romance with someone in a sober suit.

We say a lot by what we wear. Even 'I'm shy' or 'I don't want to be bothered' can be displayed by wearing clothes that make you blend in with the wallpaper. A lot of the dress messages will be subconscious — 'That's just my style' — but some very specific communication goes on too. Dress codes exist in some circles.

Using signals like handkerchiefs, gay men can suggest their interests to others. In America the AIDS fear has prompted an additional code of wearing a badge which signals only safe sexual encounters will be considered. Heterosexuals wear 'messages' too. A wedding ring or an engagement ring, for example, displays 'I'm committed'.

Self-presentation isn't only done with dress — how you wear it is also telling. Posture — how you stand, walk or sit — can speak volumes. If you cross your arms firmly across your chest, wind your legs around each other, hunch and round your shoulders, you'll look as if you feel uncomfortable and unhappy. Stand or sit straight with relaxed arms and shoulders and an easy movement of the head, and you'll feel and look more approachable. Approachability helps physical attraction, so if you want to show someone you're interested, firmly turning your back on them would be likely to give completely the wrong message.

Personality shines through too. A warm welcoming smile will get a better reception than the snarling sour-puss. Eyes are a key link, and there's much truth in the saying that the eyes are the window of the soul. Someone who won't look you in the eye may be perceived as shifty. Looks can pierce, melt, study, question. Look at someone when they're talking to you and they'll feel you're interested and listening. If you can't bring yourself to look them in the eye then concentrate on the middle of their forehead.

We give and receive a complex set of messages when we deal with other people. Because eyes and lips are recognized as two of the major means of communication, make-up is frequently used to exaggerate their prominence. Smells play their part too, a part not overlooked by commerce, and advertisers spend a great deal of time and money providing what they say are alluring scents. Actually, one of the most alluring to someone attracted to you is your own body scent. We all have our own. Obviously the smell of stale sweat isn't going to be much of a turn-on to anybody, but fresh body odours can be stimulating to a sexual partner. It's no coincidence that the base of many commercial scents is musk oil which comes from animal sex glands.

Attraction is made up of many elements, and what's attractive to others you may find repugnant. The clean-cut sporty type may make some people drool, others may go more for the academic dishevelled scruff, or the trendily dressed person about town. Women, because of social pressures, may not appreciate this variety of taste though, and feel they should try to be the ideal 'attractive' woman they see stereotyped in newspapers, magazines and so on. Those who choose women as sexual partners aren't newspapers, they're people, and people have individual taste. Some, for instance, may like the fresh-faced 'natural' look, while others like their partners to look dressed-up with lots of make-up, ready for partying. Also, what we perceive as attractive changes as we change. If you are 13 a 45-year-old seems ancient and wouldn't usually merit even a second glance. As we mature so those we're attracted to tend to be of a similar age.

After their twenties many people start panicking about age, worried that every new wrinkle is held against them in the attractiveness stakes, every grey hair a sign of decline. We live in a culture which values youthfulness, and this can lead some people to go to great extremes to stay looking young and so, to their way of thinking, attractive. Cosmetic surgery, special face creams, dyes to cover greying hair, all are taken up in the search for eternal youth. Unfortunately the result in many cases looks false, plastic and, to many people, unattractive.

We all grow old, it's a fact of life. Taking care of the body is one thing, keeping it healthy and as vibrant as possible will preserve a youthful air, but no-one can stay 20 forever, as much as they might try. Adapting to changing age, though, means adapting to loss, loss of life-span. If a person has developed an effective way of dealing with loss, they'll work through age crises. If not then they'll cling to youth, an impossible task, and the inevitability of it will begin to make them very unhappy. Remember, though, people into their 70s do fall in love, they can be attractive to others, but it's less likely if they're soured by their age rather than accept it with dignity.

For women an age crisis is often brought on by the menopause. The loss of periods signals the end of their fertility, the end of a phase of their life. Such a physical manifestation of the passing of time can throw up emotional problems, and these in turn can affect how physically well women feel.

In some countries the menopause is a cause for celebration. Needless to say this is likeliest in countries where women are forbidden much contact while they're fertile, and anyway such women will often have spent much of their fertile years pregnant. For them the menopause heralds much-welcomed freedom. In our society, however, where youth is prized, the menopause is held like a sword over women's heads, and many women suffer both physical and emotional repercussions.

What actually happens physically is that oestrogen production from the ovaries slows down and eventually stops. Hence no more ova are released, and periods may stop abruptly or become irregular before ceasing completely. Just as teenagers can be caught off-guard by mood swings induced by hormone shifts, so can menopausal women. And just as in those earlier hormone upheavals, it can be difficult to disentangle the true cause — mind or body. Mid-life, like adolescence or pregnancy, brings many changes other than the physical which need some attention.

Purely physical changes that occur at, or after, the menopause may include hot flushes and/or night sweats which can be very uncomfortable indeed. These can carry on causing discomfort for two or three years, sometimes longer. For some women hormone replacement therapy may bring relief, though it may mean having menstrual periods again. The drop in oestrogen has effects in other parts of the body, and may induce a dryness and itching everywhere, but in particular the vagina and surrounding genital area. Again hormone treatment can ease the symptoms, but water-soluble lubricants may be the first line of help for vaginal dryness.

There are metabolic changes too. The metabolism slows down, and many women around their late forties and above complain that though their eating habits haven't changed, they gain weight. An older woman's bones become more brittle. Facing such changes can be a hard task, so it's hardly surprising that many women get depressed around this time, and if it's compounded by tiredness due to waking with night sweats it's understandable that some difficulties can result, even if the rest of life is running smoothly. Having painted such a gloomy picture we should also say that many women sail through the menopause with few problems.

Men too can experience a mid-life crisis. They don't have the same physical hormone changes to contend with, but they like women may come to a stage where they re-examine their lives, and the satisfied or unfulfilled dreams of their youth. They may regret the fact that life is half-way through. Around this age offspring may leave home, which adds to the necessity of taking a new look at the parents' home and social life.

Adapting to change is one of the things we humans find hardest to do, and it often causes us anxieties. At crucial junctions in life decisions need to be made, loss accepted, gains acknowledged and conflicts resolved. If you can understand the physical changes going on in your body, and accept them, it can make it easier to identify those issues which are primarily to do with your emotional life. The body can and does affect the mind, but the reverse is also true — ignoring the needs or changes to either can lead to illness in both.

6

What Is A Good Lover?

There's no lack of advice about what makes a good lover. There are countless books, articles, radio and television programmes counselling the way to successful sex. The trouble with some of them is that if you relied only on their information you could well end up with the idea that to be a good lover you must be young, beautiful and an Olympic standard athlete. There's more to good loving than good looks and technique.

Obviously, knowing what to put where, and how to please your partner is necessary, but that's not all there is to a happy and fulfilling relationship. Once again, as so often in this book, it's important to say that there isn't a blueprint to turn you into the world's best lover. We do, though, have some ideas about what a good lover is like.

Good lovers know and appreciate their own bodies

It may surprise you to know that we've never met anyone who is completely satisfied with their own body, even if they looked as if they were perfect. It's easy for both men and women to get caught in the trap of believing that there is such a thing as a perfect body. This belief inevitably leads people to dissatisfaction, convinced they're too fat, too thin, not muscley enough, too muscley, not hairy enough, too hairy, too short, too tall. A man may worry because he believes his penis is too small, too thin, or is at the wrong angle when erect. A woman may be distressed because she feels her breasts are too large, not large enough, not equal in size; that her clitoris is too sensitive or not sensitive enough; that her vagina is too wide or not wide enough, and so on.

Part of the problem is that in the usual kind of life-style acceptable in our society there isn't much opportunity to view a range of 'normal' naked bodies. There's no point in relying on magazines which have pictures or photographs of nude men and women, since most of these are just presentations of this society's idea of perfection, and have more to do with the photographer's skill and retouching techniques than with reality. The naturist movement is still looked on as a cranky organization, and nude bathing beaches aren't exactly proliferating over Great Britain.

There are some people who haven't even seen members of their own family without clothes, so when you come to think about it, how do you know what's 'normal' and what isn't?

You'll have to take our word for it that, whatever kind of body you have, it's normal for you, and even if it doesn't match up to the photographs or diagrams you see, it's probably capable of giving you and your partner a great deal of pleasure.

In order to be a good lover you need to be familiar with and to accept your own body. If your own body frightens you, how can you share it with someone else and give them pleasure from it? You need to know what turns you on, how you like to be touched. If you can't know these things about yourself you won't be able to tell or show other people what you like.

Try standing naked in front of a full length mirror, and really look at yourself. If you're dissatisfied with what you see, ask yourself how you think you ought to be. Then think about what standards you're using to judge yourself. Whose are they? Where do they come from? Are they realistic? Are you really willing to put in the time and effort involved in making the changes if they're possible? Take a careful look at yourself. Is there any chance you might accept yourself as you actually are? Are you willing to accept that you're probably never going to be any taller or shorter than you are now, that your eyes will remain the same distance apart, that your bone structure won't alter? Are you willing to accept that there are some things you cannot change, unless of course you're prepared to spend enormous amounts of time and money, and have some extraordinary operations? There may be small changes you can make, good points you can highlight, but do be careful, once again, not to feel that you're not acceptable if you're not perfect — no-one else is either, and it probably doesn't put you off them.

Good lovers love touch

Sex is ever present in our daily lives. It would be virtually impossible to go through a day without being made aware of it through the media, jokes, advertisements and so on. Sensuality, though, isn't so acceptable, and yet the greatest pleasures in sexual contact are experienced through the senses, especially the sense of touch. A good lover doesn't judge sexual success by an orgasm score, but by the quality of the pleasure both people experience.

In our society there are strong taboos about people touching each other, yet we know that cuddles, hugs and strokes are necessary for healthy development. There's a great deal of research proving that babies who don't get hugs and kisses from their parents don't develop normally, and some have serious emotional problems. In our early months of life how we're touched will have a great influence on the way we approach life. Most parents seem to understand this intuitively, and most babies get a lot of loving physical contact. The blocks come on as we grow up and this contact is withdrawn or rationed. After our first few years of life, the number of people who we can touch, and who can touch us, are severely limited. In our culture even a touch on the arm can make people shy away.

We learn the rules about touch by hearing such things as, 'Don't touch that, you'll break it', 'Don't touch this or you'll get hurt', 'Don't touch yourself there, it's naughty', 'You mustn't touch people like that, they don't like it'. Some of these rules are for our own safety, some are social guidance, but both come over as instructions. Similarly, if we don't see people around us touching each other we're likely to make the deduction that this is out of bounds, and we take our social instruction from their example. Many people grow up never having seen their parents hug, hold hands or kiss, or show much physical affection, and yet this is one of the most important lessons parents could teach their children. Little boys, particularly, are often deprived of physical contact very early on — kissing and cuddling doesn't fit in to people's idea of a 'real man', so boys may be taught such behaviour is cissy.

Children can also be given a message that touching is specifically to do with sex, and is 'naughty'. Quite often if parents are caught cuddling they get embarrassed about it, or it's something they only do in their bedroom where the children may be forbidden from disturbing them. Anyone who watches television (and most children do!) will soon believe that hugging and kissing usually lead to sex. All this fosters the idea that touching is sexual. And this leads to the inhibitions many of us grow up with about physical contact — we daren't touch someone in case they misunderstand our motives.

The problem that this gives us in our sex lives is that since touching isn't seen as something which of itself can be an expression of love, it can't be indulged in unless it's going to end in intercourse. Yet the need for physical contact which we had as a baby doesn't disappear as we grow up, even though the opportunities for getting as much as we need do shrink. Most boys learn that physical contact is only legitimate through sport (football, rugby, wrestling etc) and sex. Girls are often more fortunate in that's it's seen as all right for them to cuddle and be cuddled — they'll see female relatives, for instance, kiss and hug far more often than boys will see their male relatives behave similarly. So women are less likely to be so dependent on sex for physical closeness.

Good lovers enjoy touching and being touched not only as a prelude to love-making, but for the sheer sensual pleasure of stroking and caressing.

One start to increasing your own knowledge and experience in the pleasures of touch is to give yourself about half-an-hour when you can be alone and in a comfortable place. Get undressed, lie or sit down. Using some body lotion or massage oil, gently stroke yourself, concentrating on parts of your body you can easily reach — hands, arms, legs, feet, torso. Include your genitals if you wish, but it's not necessary to concentrate on them. It's a myth that sensual pleasure can only be experienced through our genitals — the whole body is capable of giving you and your partner erotic and sensual pleasure. While you massage and caress yourself, stay aware of what it feels like, and become conscious of what kind of touch you most like — soft, firm, fingertips, nails, slow, vigorous — and where you most like to be touched.

This suggestion isn't intended as an exercise in sexual arousal, though this may happen. If it does, just enjoy it. The main purpose of taking time like this is to get to know yourself. As you learn what you like, you'll also be learning how to share this with a partner.

Good lovers have fun

There are hundreds of ways of pleasing and being pleased by a sexual partner, but none of them will happen unless you enjoy touching and being touched. One of the best things about sex is that it can be such fun. It's one of the ways that adults can get to play, to act out fantasies, and be a child again. Serious passion has its place, but so does child-like pleasure and a good laugh. Sometimes you may try something new and it doesn't work — if you can see the funny side of the fact that you've been hooked together by your teeth braces, or get cramp when your partner is at the peak of passion, then it can save you torturing yourself by seeing things as 'failure' when they're no such thing.

Good lovers are adventurous

Sex can be pretty boring if it becomes routine and predictable. Trying something new can bring fresh excitement — making love in the afternoon maybe, or in a different room, different positions, genital kissing or, if you like, hanging from the chandeliers. In private who but the pair of you need care if you try different clothes and act out each other's fantasies?

Good lovers love loving

What we mean by loving is a sense of commitment to another person based on mutual affection and a desire to care for each other. It's perfectly possible to have sex with someone you don't love, or even really know, and have an enjoyable experience. However, that kind of experience can't honestly be compared to making love with someone for whom you care a great deal. Alex Comfort, author of *The Joy of Sex*, compares sex without love to cooking without heat. Good lovers treat each other as whole people, not merely objects of desire and gratification. They are sensitive to their partner's needs and wishes and will want to respond to them.

Good lovers relax

If you're tense, uptight and inhibited, you'll have great difficulty pleasing someone else, because you'll be too concerned about your own anxieties. Relax — after all, this is meant to be pleasure, not an exam or a competition. Sensuality is virtually impossible if you can't relax. If you're making love with someone for the first time of course you'll be nervous and excited, and so it's a good idea to spend quite a bit of time stroking, kissing and soothing away that nervousness. If someone is incredibly tense it can have physical repercussions which actually prevent love-making, such as lack of erection or vaginal dryness or muscular spasm, which in turn can make the person believe they're a 'failure', so they get anxious about 'failure' and worry that it might happen again, which leaves them tense, and so a vicious circle begins. Relax!

Good lovers talk about it

Imagine that a group of Martians come to Earth on a fact-finding mission. They know nothing about our culture, but want to understand it. Sex would certainly confuse them. They could reasonably assume our society was obsessed with sex, since they'd notice the many books, films, plays, songs, adverts and jokes that had sex as their main theme. They'd also notice, though, that not many people talk openly about it, resorting to innuendo, nudge-nudge joking and coy embarrassed references.

Discussing sex, particularly if things are going wrong, is very important. Lack of communication can make things worse. Here are some examples of how that might happen:

> Anita has a new boyfriend. She enjoys his company, and they have many things in common, but she doesn't like the way he always wants to have physical contact with her in public, holding her arm, putting his arm around her shoulders. When they're alone he kisses and caresses her more than she wants and she finds his need for closeness overwhelming. She deals with this by avoiding physical contact by pulling away from him or pushing him away. He interprets this as a 'come-on' and believes that she wants him to try even harder — so he does.
>
> John and Geoff have lived together for several years. Each feels their sex life has become routine and boring. Neither likes to talk to the other about their feelings in case it hurts the other. However, they have become irritable and short-tempered, and argue about trivial domestic details. John is beginning to find other men attractive and is contemplating starting an affair. Geoff senses this and feels rejected.
>
> One afternoon Tom says to his wife, 'Isn't it lovely! The children are out and we have the house to ourselves.' His wife smiles and nods and returns to her reading. Tom was actually wanting to make love, but the sexual invitation went unnoticed. In his mind this confirmed his feeling that his wife was disinterested in sex.

It is as important to talk about sex as it is about anything else. Without talking, misunderstandings can easily arise and needs go unmet simply through lack of asking.

To help clarify your thoughts and feelings about sex and what you want to say to your partner, think about what you do and don't enjoy.

Write down any beliefs and fears that make you hesitate to talk with your partner.

There are sets of beliefs which make it difficult for people to talk openly about their sexual needs — here are some examples.

1. Sex is mystical and wonderful — talking will spoil it Think for a moment about anything you think is wonderful and beautiful: a rose, a work of art, a delicious meal, particular music, an intricate machine. If it were true that talking about something wonderful spoiled it, then there would be no music scores, no gardening books, no gourmet recipes, no art classes. In fact it's generally agreed that discussing a piece of music, or a good meal, actually enhances the experience rather than spoils it. Why should sex be any different?

2. Sex should come naturally Sex is a biological process, and animals seem to organize their sex lives without too many problems. Human beings, however, aren't born knowing how to be good lovers. The instinct and drive are there, but to be a pleasurable experience it needs rather more thought than a purely biological act as practised by animals. As making love is regarded as an opportunity to give and receive mutual pleasure, how can you do that if you don't know what might please your partner? Perfect, spontaneous, sex is an attractive notion, and it's certainly part of the romantic fantasy, but anyone who believes in this idea won't be able to deal with problems when they arise, which they almost inevitably will.

3. Sex should be good all the time When two people are first attracted to each other everything they do pleases the other. Each wants the other's approval. Differences and problems are suppressed in the excitement. As time passes, and the first excitement dies down, things which may have been ignored begin to make themselves felt. There may be a difference in sexual preferences, or anxieties about other aspects of life. Sex is only part of our lives, there are a lot of other things which also demand our attention and time — jobs, finance and family may all be pressing. Preoccupations relating to these aspects of life can interfere with sex.

Just as sometimes you may go off food, so you may go off sex for a while, or experience impotence or lack of orgasm. The romantically-minded may panic and believe these are signs the magic has gone and that there's something essentially wrong with the relationship. The sensible thing to do in these circumstances is to share with your partner whatever you're thinking and feeling. You may fear doing so, worrying that your partner will take it as a sign of rejection. If you tell someone that it's not them personally you're rejecting, but rather something you're worrying about he or she stands a chance of understanding what's happening and not be left to guess and perhaps jump to inaccurate conclusions.

Beware of overdoing this, however. Sometimes you may feel 'turned-off', or be unable to maintain an erection, or experience premature ejaculation, or not reach orgasm for no apparent reason. If this is an isolated event it's probably best to just accept it and pass on, just as a good cook accepts that on occasions the souffle will fail to rise and there's no point agonizing over it. Going over and over such events in your mind, or with your partner, is only likely to increase anxiety. Human beings aren't sex-robots, ever willing and able to perform once the right buttons are pressed. If it's a continuing problem or block it's worth discussion, but avoid sexual hypochondria.

Make a list of any external factors which might affect your sex life, for example problems at work, money, in-laws, ill-health, children and tiredness.

4. If someone really loves you, they'll know how to please you This is the mind-reading trap again. Don't assume your partner is a telepathy expert, or that if they can't read your mind it means they don't love or want you. You may be worried that if you ask for something different the other person will think you are demanding, selfish or even perverted. Of course there's always the risk that is just what they will think, and they will go on to reject you. However, if you don't communicate with them your chance of sexual happiness, as you see it, is limited. There's a risk either way. Another fear is that your partner might do what you want just because you asked, without really wanting to. So it's vital that each takes responsibility for setting their own personal limits, and allows each other the opportunity and freedom of saying no.

If you're sexually involved with someone at the moment, was there a time when your sex life with your partner was better than it is now? If so, what's different? Think about the things which might have been, or are contributing to the change. Is there anything you have done, or not done, that's causing the change?

5. *Good lovers want the same things* There are bound to be times in any long-term relationship when differences occur. The inevitable temptation is to avoid conflicts which can arise as a result of different wishes and expectations. If you submit to that temptation and don't communicate directly about differences of opinion or need, then you risk increasing feelings or resentment and frustration, both for you and your partner.

In an earlier exercise we suggested that you listed fears that might stop you speaking honestly to your partner. What were they? Is it that they'll react negatively, or that you feel guilty and have no right to ask for something different? Guilt has a way of bunging a spoke in the works of any kind of communication. In order to avoid the paralysis guilt can provoke, think assertively, and accept that you have every right to your own thoughts, feelings, preferences and desires. You also have the right to tell people about them. They have the same rights, and so are entitled to say no if they wish. Guilt has no part in that communication.

What if . . .

What if you meet with a refusal of your requests? You can accept it, or you can try to find out what's behind the refusal. Which you choose to do depends on how important the issue is for you.

If you do decide to look further at the reasons for the refusal, you could discover some fantasy fears influencing your partner's response. For example 'If I wear sexy underwear, you'll think I'm a tart', 'If I tell you my fantasies you'll think I'm perverted', 'Masturbation isn't good, it isn't *real* sex'. If you do uncover such fears, you can begin to address them. Or you may reveal some hidden resentments that are causing the refusal. For example, 'Why should I take more time when you never take the initiative?' 'Whenever I ask you for something you say no, and now you expect me to change to suit you.'

You may not relish hearing such criticisms, but it may be worth it in the long run. The more you talk, however difficult that is, and however much the words may seem to stick in your throat at times, the more chance there is of finding ways to ensure the relationship grows rather than stagnates.

The guidelines for good communication about sex are the same as for any other matter:

1. Be clear about what you think, feel and want.
2. Be positive — talk about what you like and phrase what you don't want positively. For instance, try using 'and' instead of 'but' — 'I know that you'd like to do such-and-such, and while I'm not keen I would like some change.'
3. Be responsible for yourself — don't accuse the other person for your reactions.
4. Be specific — avoid generalizations.
5. Be willing to experiment, unless what your partner asks goes completely against your wishes.

Rising passion

Making love can begin in any number of ways. It may be playful, tender, seductive, or even follow an argument. Generally though, the aim is to give and receive pleasure. While quick, passionate sex may have some rewards, there's little doubt that savouring the experience, as you would a good meal, is the most satisfying. The process of arousal to passion is a pleasure in itself.

Foreplay, as it's rather technically known, may begin with the eyes. A long, lingering look can make the skin tingle. Watching someone undress or undressing them can be a feast for the eyes and get hormones triggering off other responses. The heartbeat seems louder, the breathing faster. As lovers move closer the other person's smell may be a further attraction. All the senses get on the alert. Touch is the most powerful. Passionate kissing, nibbling with the lips, butterfly kisses on the body, exploring hands on parts of the body that no-one other than a lover is allowed to caress all add to the excitement for both. Some people like firm touching, others gentle. Some people like both, but at different times.

A good lover doesn't just go for the obvious. There are numerous erogenous zones on the body and a good lover will know that feet are highly sexy for some people, others may adore having the crook of their elbow gently tickled, or their neck kissed or massaged, their inner thigh caressed, their back scratched, or their head massaged. The whole body is sexual, not just the genitals.

There may be times when foreplay of itself is sufficient pleasure, it needn't necessarily lead into another phase. If the sexual charge is high though, passion gets unreined and the body wants more.

In readiness Both sexes have quite obvious physical changes which happen during arousal. Women's nipples become erect, and their breasts may increase in size. Blood gets pumped to the breasts, making the veins prominent, and to the pelvic region, causing several changes. One of the first things women notice when they're sexually excited is a moistness coming from their vagina. This moisture seeps through the vaginal walls and is necessary to aid penetration and stimulation of the clitoris. The rush of blood increases the size of the clitoris, swells the labia minora (inner lips) and causes the labia majora (outer lips) to spread flatter. The vagina gets in readiness by expanding, and it becomes both wider and longer as the uterus and cervix pull away.

When men are sexually excited blood rushes into the spongy tissue of the penis, making it stiff and longer. With the erection the scrotum thickens and the testes draw closer to the body. Like women, many men may find their nipples become erect too.

Wanting more From foreplay and arousal, we move to what's known as the plateau phase. Women's breasts continue to enlarge and the areolae around the nipple swell. In both sexes the chest, back and abdomen may come out in a sort of pink sex blush. Whether or not there's penetration from a penis, the bottom third of the vagina closes up a bit in order to grip a penis while its upper part continues to expand. The clitoris retreats into its hood. The heat generated from two sexually excited exploring bodies can bring both partners out into quite a sweat.

While men's bodies flush pink, their penis tip may also change colour to a purplish red. The tip swells, as do the testes, which are still drawing closer to the body. The foreskin retracts as the diameter of the penis increases, and a man may experience contractions of the muscles in the rectum.

Sheer bliss Nearing an orgasm can be like waiting for a sneeze that you know will be a satisfying relief. In both sexes the increasing urgency can be heard in the heavier breathing, perhaps accompanied by sighs or groans, and seen in the eyes as the pupils expand. The nostrils flare. The cords in the neck stand out. All the muscles in the body seem tense as it rhythmically nears a climax.

Orgasm involves the whole body, even though the peak of the experience centres on the genitals. A climax causes muscular spasms which in the male prompt ejaculation of the semen, perhaps three or four bursts, and in the female both the uterus and the lower third of the vagina have waves of rhythmic contractions. Just like a huge sneeze, an orgasm seems to explode in the head too, and it has been known for people actually to lose consciousness at this point.

Rarely do a couple climax together. On some occasions one partner may not come to orgasm at all and not be too worried about it, while on other occasions they may want their satisfied partner to pay them a little more physical attention, and not roll over and drift into contented sleep until they too have enjoyed a climax.

In the afterglow Everything quietens down now the passion has been satiated. The technical name for this is the resolution phase. A couple may feel particularly close now, though perhaps a little chilly if they're unclothed as their sex flush subsides. Blood that's rushed to the main areas of excitement is dissipated. The penis returns to its flaccid state, the areolae subside, leaving the nipples prominent, and the vaginal contractions fade. Within seconds of orgasm the clitoris resumes its normal size, but the uterus, cervix and vagina may take half an hour to return to normal.

Enjoying yourself

There are other ways to come to orgasm than through penetration of a penis in a vagina. In fact for many women only direct stimulation of the clitoris ever achieves orgasm. Masturbation is something many people try out at an early age. Even tiny children get pleasure from touching their genitals, and the young teenager may discover the delights of rhythmically rubbing their penis or clitoris until they climax.

Guilt may colour their pleasure, though, if their parents, religion, or other formative sources have decreed masturbation to be disgusting, self-abuse and sinful. Some may fear they're doing themselves harm if they've taken in myths about it making you go blind or damaging the genitals in some way. Self-awareness and self-exploration are rarely, if ever, harmful. If someone compulsively masturbates then they are either bored or emotionally ill. Masturbation of itself isn't wrong, but any compulsion warrants attention. Knowing how your own body reacts to sexual arousal and how you like to be touched are advantages in becoming part of a loving partnership.

Some people like the addition of sex toys such as vibrators or dildos (penis substitutes) for solo sexual pleasure, or to add to the variety in a sexual partnership.

Try something different

If you had baked beans on toast three or four times a week you might get pretty bored with the taste and even the sight of them. If you make love exactly the same way two or three times a week for years then you'll get pretty bored with that too. You can experiment with all sorts of positions, building up your sexual repertoire, and this applies to masturbation too. It doesn't always have to be at night, in bed and unclothed for a start. Particular clothing may be a real turn-on for some people. Perhaps your partner would relish finding you in sexy underwear, or would like to make love fully clothed, while at other times wanting naked skin contact. Use your imagination as you do to present interesting meals. There are a few basic recipes though which you can use to work from.

- ***Mutual masturbation*** Love-making doesn't have to include penetration at all. Masturbating each other by hand or using sex toys or whatever can be as enjoyable. Homosexual couples may regularly use this type of love-making.

- ***Missionary position*** This is perhaps the most famous position where, for heterosexual couples, the woman lies on her back with the man on top of her. This isn't limitless, though, as the partner underneath can change the position by moving her legs together, apart, round her partner's back or over his shoulders, and the man on top can also change position.

- ***Woman superior*** Here the female partner is on top. She can move into many different positions from there, such as choosing to lie or sit astride being just two.

- ***Back to front*** Pregnant women can find this position particularly suitable as if their partner approaches them from behind there's no pressure on the 'bump'. This back to front position can be tried lying down, side by side, kneeling or even standing.

- ***Props*** You don't always have to make love on a bed. Sometimes making love on the floor of the living room or kitchen may be an extra turn on. One partner might sit on a chair with their partner astride them, or kneel on the floor while their partner lies with their legs over the edge of the bed. You could use a pillow under the small of the back, turn the lights on, leave them off, have soft music, soul music or complete silence. There are numerous possibilities. Use the props around you to add to your sexual variety.

- ***Oral sex*** This doesn't mean talking about it. It means using your mouth and tongue to stimulate your partner's genitals by kissing, licking and sucking.

- ***Anal sex*** Penetration of the anus by a penis can cause some damage to the rectum, and hence add to any risk of AIDS. It is a common practice in some cultures and is often practised by homosexual men or heterosexuals who are curious about it (although in Britain heterosexual anal sex is illegal). Oral or vaginal sex should never follow on from anal intercourse without first washing.

Making love involves two people. No sexual variation should be tried if one partner has strong objections to it. Saying no is difficult if you are afraid of being thought of as prudish, unloving or selfish; or if you fear the other person may leave you if you refuse to go along with what they want.

Don't let these difficulties stop you — you have an absolute right to decide what to do with your body. You can say something like, 'I like being with you, but I'm not enjoying what we're doing and I want to stop', or 'I'm afraid you'll think I'm a prude, or that I don't love you (or whatever it is that you are afraid of), but I don't want to carry on doing this', or 'No, I don't want you to do that, but I'd love it if you'd. . . .', or just, 'No!'

If your partner ignores you, or tries to persuade you to change your mind you have every right to be angry at that discounting of your wishes. There are choices open to you — you may leave the relationship altogether if you don't want to continue being with someone who is so disrespectful towards you, or you can decide to discuss the matter so that you understand each other better.

If you decide to talk about it, you could use the formula we describe in chapter 4 as a way of starting off. For example, 'I like the relationship we have together, but there is one thing that I am unhappy about. I know you enjoy oral sex but when I say that I don't want to do that you carry on as though I hadn't said anything. (*Reporting*) I feel angry that you discount me this way, and worried that you think I'm strait-laced and prudish. I don't think I am, but this is something that I just don't like. (*Relating*) I'd like you to stop ignoring me (*Requesting*). I'll enjoy our love-making much more if I feel that you care about what I want. (*Result*)'

One choice that we don't recommend is that you allow your own wishes to be overridden, and agree to do things that you don't really want to do. You may solve one of your problems (that is, avoiding saying no) in the short-term, but the relationship as a whole will suffer in the long-term.

How often?

Sex drive, otherwise known as libido, is an extremely variable phenomenon. It's an appetite, and like other appetites varies from individual to individual and also depends upon what mood and physical shape they're in. It can change during a menstrual cycle for women, perhaps with peaks at either ovulation or pre-period. It can be altered by the weather — 'It's too hot and sticky' — by events — 'I'm too upset and tired' — by the mood in the relationship — 'I love you so much now I want to show it'.

Fertility specialists recommend that if you want to get pregnant you should make love two to four times a week so you won't miss ovulation, and they feel this won't put a strain on most couples' relationships. However, some couples may make love once a week, once a fortnight or every few months, and are perfectly happy with that, while others want passionate love-making every day. Couples may go through patches where one or the other doesn't much feel like making love. If outside pressures are taking their toll then a partner may understand and be prepared to tolerate the situation, but if loss of libido signals a problem in the relationship then it needs talking about. Making love can mend arguments, but only if both partners want the mend.

7
What Can Go Wrong With Sex?

Sex can go wrong. When it does its importance can get out of perspective in a relationship, souring other aspects and becoming the vital but unattainable satisfaction.

No-one is a sex machine, able to turn on or off whatever else may be happening in their lives, and a person's sex drive, or libido, will hit perfectly natural highs and lows. If these don't coincide with a partner's then there may be a bit of explaining and reassuring to do, but it shouldn't become a major problem unless the partner is completely self-centred.

As we said in the previous chapter, there is no such thing as a 'recommended' or 'healthy' frequency to make love. Of course if two people of varying libido get together they will need to work out a compromise if both are to remain contented and not feel either deprived or pressured. Pressure or misgivings about sexual relationships can trigger many of what are referred to as psycho-sexual disorders, where a person's feelings have a direct physical effect on their sexuality.

Lost the urge When one of a couple doesn't feel like making love for a long time it can begin to put pressure on the relationship. Sometimes the reason the person doesn't feel like it is because they have a grudge against their partner for some reason, an outstanding problem to sort out which, consciously or not, is expressed by withdrawing from intimate physical contact. If loss of libido has been caused by other problems in the relationship then it's those which need sorting out before the sex drive will return. Often, though, it's simply that some of the enjoyment seems to have gone, perhaps love-making has become mundane, too predictable or too orgasm-orientated.

If the trouble is simply that the pleasure has gone flat then it can help to actually ban intercourse for an agreed period — three weeks, three months, or whatever you decide between you. During that time you can still enjoy each other's bodies but in a different way. It's back to basics time, but very enjoyable basics — touching, stroking, kissing and massage. The idea is to awaken the pleasure a body can get from its entire skin surface, to show the pleasure that can be received from caring attention.

Too often people only try to make love, or kiss and cuddle when it's time for bed and both are tired. It can be soothing to drift off to sleep after making love, but if you're exhausted, and all you want to do is sleep, then the physical exertion of sex may seem like a pressure rather than a pleasure. So if the sensual stroking and massage are to have beneficial effects it's best if neither partner is too tired to bother.

The things you need are a warm room, a bath towel, some oil or massage lotion, and warm hands. Spend as much time as you like — hours if you feel like it. One partner should massage/stroke/kiss the other all over, starting at the feet or hands and working all over, though avoiding the genital area or female breasts. The lucky beneficiary should say what feels particularly pleasant, or unpleasant, and so encourage their partner to please them. Then the place on the bath towel should be reversed and the other partner become the recipient of some sensual stroking.

After as many sessions as the couple want, the stroking can increase to include the breasts and genitals, and even mutual masturbation, but still not full intercourse. This technique, known as sensate focus, can rekindle a couple's passion as well as educate them on what their partner really likes, when they otherwise might have relied on guesswork or misguided assumptions. At the end of the agreed abstinence from sex with penetration the couple can resume full intercourse. If they wish they can retain some of the techniques they discovered during their sensual explorations.

How can anyone fancy my body? Satisfying love-making isn't dependent on physical perfection. This is just as well, as no-one's perfect and most of us have parts of our body we wish something would reach and reshape. Countless women, though, will only make love in the dark because they feel ashamed to let their partners see what they consider to be abnormalities. They may be worried about their breasts being too small, too big, having an inverted nipple, a little body hair, drooping breasts, one larger than the other. All these things are perfectly normal, but they don't think so. They may think that their genitals are abnormal, that their labia minora (inner lips) are too big, that they're too hairy — you name it, someone will worry about.

Men, too, suffer anxiety, usually about their penis size or shape. As much as men are told that penis size doesn't matter, they take some convincing. It's almost as if it were some kind of competition, but it's honestly true that what a man does with his penis (and the rest of his body) is far more important than its size. A man might also worry if his penis goes at what he considers to be a peculiar angle when erect — again, though, this isn't likely to present any problems, except for his own anxiety levels.

These anxieties, especially if they're such a cause of embarrassment that they're not expressed, can cause problems for the other partner. If someone is holding back, human nature being the way it is, the other partner will probably think it's is something to do with them — that they're not good enough, not sexy enough, not fanciable. Hence all sorts of unspoken barriers can go up, when often there's no need at all.

It hurts Pain on intercourse in either sex should be investigated. It can signal infection or other medical problems requiring attention. In some women it can be a symptom of an emotional problem, but more of that in 'Sex is impossible' (page 123).

No orgasm The first thing to say here is that enjoyable love-making doesn't always have to culminate in orgasm. One partner may decide to devote themself on a particular occasion to their partner's pleasure and get satisfaction from that. However, if one partner never achieves a climax it can be frustrating for them both, and could signal a problem. Women are generally thought to be the ones to suffer lack of orgasm, but men, too, can be unable to climax or take a very long time about it.

Sometimes the problem is as basic as not paying enough attention to arousal or continued stimulation. Women often don't climax purely through intercourse. Though enjoying penetration they may get greater pleasure from rhythmic stimulation of the clitoris, and if their partner hasn't cottoned on to this, or she hasn't told him, then it could be a simple remedy to lack of orgasm. If a woman's partner suffers from premature ejaculation their love-making may be all over before she's really got into the mood so her climax will also be affected. There are people though who, even with a caring and attentive partner, just cannot let go, cannot hit a peak whilst making love.

Because orgasm involves surrendering yourself to physical sensation, some people may be worried that they will look daft, that their facial contortions will put the other person off, that groaning or panting will be heard by others. Any of these things, if taken to heart, can be enough to put someone off and make them hold back. Loss of control can be frightening too. In orgasm we are vulnerable, and it's a very intimate moment. That intimacy terrifies some people because they fear being overwhelmed or losing themselves.

If someone has been taught that sex is somehow disgusting and shameful and that their own body should be censored, perhaps even from their own eyes, then understandably they may have reservations about giving physical expression to sexual desires and let someone else in on their 'shameful' bits. Men and women are sometimes taught that perfectly ordinary love-making can do damage to a woman, and a misguided fear of that can be a severe inhibitor. Such deep-seated anxieties and sexual guilt may be eased by a very understanding, patient, and giving partner. Sometimes, though, the process can be helped by a sex therapist.

Lastly, if there are problems in a relationship, if there's any resentment or anger stewing, then it's quite likely that love-making will be affected, sometimes by one partner withholding the satisfaction of orgasm.

Sex is impossible Both sexes can be struck by an inability to make love at all. Most men, at some time in their life, find that they are unable to get or maintain an erection, often for no particular reason, or at least not one to cause continuing problems. Usually it's nothing to worry about and normal 'service' resumes. If a man gets overly anxious about an incident of impotence then this of itself can become the cause of further episodes. Pressure from a sexual partner may also bring on performance anxiety and in turn cause impotence.

The most common cause of impotence is emotional. There are some physical causes — some drugs, for instance, can have adverse effects on a person's sexual ability, so if in doubt you should consult a doctor. Alcohol has a well-earned reputation for rousing the passion but paralysing the means, so that too can be a culprit. But in the majority of cases prolonged impotence is a sign of some inner unresolved problems. A sympathetic partner may help break through such barriers, but, again, sex therapy can be beneficial.

Women often think there's a physical problem when they find they're unable to make love. A common fear is that their vagina is too small, or that sex will inevitably be painful, so they freeze. Because love-making for a woman involves allowing someone inside her, that can ring a whole lot of alarm bells, and be terrifying.

That terror can cause the vaginal muscles to clamp so tightly that nothing is allowed in. Sometimes the terror is so great that the woman can't even touch herself, or use tampons. This fear and its physical repercussions are known as vaginismus — a physical barrier with an emotional core.

Self-help can be useful here. If the root cause of vaginismus is a fear of a woman's own body, then teaching herself to look (with the aid of a mirror), feel, examine, learn about and accept herself may dissolve the fear. If self-examination is physically painful then this may be due to lack of lubrication (caused by anxiety) and using a water-soluble lubricant (such as K-Y Jelly or Senselle) can solve that problem. Talking to other women can be immensely reassuring. A gentle, patient, caring, and truly seductive partner can help through this problem. Talking to a sex therapist may help lay some sexual ghosts and open up the prospect of sexual enjoyment.

Just occasionally sex being impossible for a woman has a physical cause. If the hymen, the piece of skin-like substance across the entry to the vagina, is unusually thick and completely covers the entrance to the vagina then medical intervention may be necessary to break it. It's rare for it to cause problems though, as generally it's incomplete, or so thin that it's broken before or at first sexual intercourse, without any noticeable effect except perhaps a slight show of blood.

Over too quickly Women may reach orgasm quickly, but if they do, it doesn't mean that they can't carry on making love to their partner if they wish. If a man ejaculates very quickly this can leave his partner frustrated and both of them upset. Premature ejaculation is a very common problem — premature meaning within two minutes of penetration — and completely outside the male's control. Inexperience, over-excitement and nervousness may all play their part in the problem and so there's a great deal that self-help can do to delay the moment of climax.

If a man is able to make love for a second time after he's ejaculated (allowing for a recovery period), then this second arousal may not be felt quite so intensely and so allow more relaxed love-making. Wearing a fairly thick condom may lessen intensity and so encourage a longer build-up to climax. Turning his mind to some other fairly mundane thought may aid control.

A method which requires a loving and committed partner to help is called the squeeze technique. The aim is for the man to become aware of the feelings in his penis and so be able to stop before climax, with the help of his partner, and then carry on and again stop before climax. His partner helps by squeezing just below the head of the penis, using thumb and two fingers, for about 15 seconds, starting when the man senses he's close to orgasm. The couple can use this technique during mutual masturbation, or during full love-making, though when you're first trying the technique it's probably easiest in masturbation. Over a period of time the squeeze technique will help the man gain more self control over his love-making. No man has complete control over climax, but it can be increased.

Physical obstacles Making love, though desired, may be difficult for some people if their general mobility is impaired. It doesn't mean sex is impossible, but it may help to seek expert advice on positions and so on which may make things easier. A strategically placed pillow may ease a bad back, for instance. People with severe disabilities may be helped by specialist advice and perhaps the use of some sex aids. An organization called SPOD (Sexual and Personal Relationship Problems of the Disabled) have a range of leaflets available as well as individual advice if required.

8

Keeping Sexual Health

Making love means taking decisions. The first is whether or not you want to. If you're heterosexual then the second decision is likely to be whether or not you wish to get pregnant. If you don't then you must either avoid sex or take precautions. For both heterosexuals and homosexuals, if this is a new partner, or you're not in a long-term monogamous relationship, then you also need to decide if and how you want to protect your health in this encounter.

To make these last two decisions, about contraception and/or health, you need information on the options.

Birth Control

The perfect method of birth control hasn't been discovered. Each method has advantages and disadvantages. A woman's medical history is an important consideration, and specialist advice and birth control supplies are available free from family planning clinics. There are also specialist youth advisory centres in some areas. In the UK most GPs also provide a free birth control service, though they cannot prescribe condoms or the contraceptive sponge, and it may also be harder to get advice from them on natural family planning methods. Let's take a look at the main pros and cons of all the generally available contraceptives.

The Pill

How it works: There are two main types of contraceptive pill — the combined pill (containing oestrogen and progestogen), and the progestogen-only pill which is sometimes referred to as the mini-pill. The combined pill, which is generally taken for 21 days out of every 28, prevents the follicles from releasing an egg and creates a change in the mucous around the cervix, making it hostile to sperm. The progestogen-only pill relies just on creating this mucus around the cervix to prevent sperm from entering the womb, and these pills are taken continuously.

Combined pills come in varying dosages, high (which is no longer used for contraceptive purposes), medium and low dose. This refers to the content of oestrogen and most users these days are on low or medium. There are also what are known as triphasic and biphasic pills. Triphasic pills try to imitate closely the body's own cycle by breaking into three different dosages of hormone in the course of one packet, and biphasic use two. Both mean that overall less hormone is administered than in standard combined pills.

Advantages: The combined pill is about 93–99.9% effective in preventing pregnancy when taken exactly as instructed. The hormone action which prevents ovulation also means that the lining of the womb, the endometrium, doesn't build up as much during the cycle, hence the pill can ease some period problems such as pain or heavy bleeding. The increase in oestrogen means that some skin conditions, such as acne, can benefit. It provides a protective effect against ovarian and endometrical cancer. The pill does not quash sexual spontaneity, it's not messy and so suits many people who are squeamish about their bodies.

The progestogen-only pill's advantage over the combined is that it doesn't carry a risk of thrombosis. It's about 96–98% effective.

Disadvantages: The combined pill can be a contributory factor in thrombosis and strokes. If a woman is overweight and/or smokes, especially if she's nearing 35, she may be advised against this pill. She may be similarly warned off if she has a personal (or sometimes even family) history of thrombosis, high blood pressure, crescendo migraine, heart problems occurring at a young age, diabetes or liver disease. There seems to be an increased risk of cervical cancer in pill users, though the pill may be one of many factors involved. Some people on the pill complain of headaches, weight gain, loss of libido, irregular bleeding or a deterioration in a skin condition and these may make them reconsider. Often such side-effects can be sorted out by a change of pill, but sometimes it's necessary to choose an alternative method.

Contraceptive failure on the combined pill is usually due to missing a pill or losing the effect of one through sickness, severe diarrhoea, or taking anti-biotics or some other drugs, as these can seriously reduce the pill's effectiveness. In some cases when a woman stops taking the pill there's a break before return to her natural cycle, though this generally disappears within six months and rarely lasts longer than two years. Hormone treatment to push the ovaries into action again can sometimes rectify that 'hangover' effect if pregnancy is desired.

The progestogen-only pill can cause irregular bleeding which to some women is distressing. It can also cause a complete lack of periods, and this, too, can lead to worry about whether or not conception might have taken place. Some women get cysts on their ovaries whilst taking this pill. If the progestogen-only pill fails then there is an increased risk of ectopic pregnancy. This is a dangerous condition, where the fertilized egg embeds itself outside the womb, usually in the fallopian tubes. Any history of ectopic pregnancies rules out a woman from taking this pill.

The Condom (sheath/rubber/johnnie/french letter)

How it works: The condom has a very simple, yet effective way of working. It contains the sperm upon ejaculation. Some condoms are also coated with spermicide or can be used with spermicidal pessaries for maximum efficiency.

Advantages: There are few health side-effects to condom usage except for the rare person who suffers a rubber allergy, and even then there are special brands available to cater for this need. As a contraceptive it is about 85–98% effective, and it also offers some health protection. Because of the barrier it presents it can help to prevent the transmission of certain diseases, and is especially valuable in guarding against cervical cancer and the virus HIV which causes AIDS (see pp. 136–137).

It's likely that people will use a condom as a health protection measure along with another method of birth control if pregnancy would be a disaster. You don't need to see a doctor to get condoms. You can buy them in chemists or from slot machines in some toilets, or they can be obtained free from family planning clinics.

Disadvantages: As the condom must be put on an erect penis it can interfere with sexual spontaneity, but this may be a small price to pay. Men have often complained that condoms reduce sensitivity, but there are are finer brands on the market, and for some men, reducing sensitivity may help with a problem such as premature ejaculation. Great care must be taken not to split the rubber with torn fingernails, and also that it's withdrawn intact from the vagina before the penis becomes flaccid.

The Cap (diaphragm, cervical cap, vault cap and vimule)

How it works: There are various types of cap, but the most commonly used is the diaphragm. The cap, like the condom, acts as a barrier. In this case, though, the woman inserts it before intercourse, well beforehand if she wants to. The diaphragm covers the cervix, and wedges behind the pubic bone. Cervical caps are smaller and merely cover the cervix. It's always been advised that the cap should be used with spermicide, usually cream, and topped up with a pessary if love-making takes place more than three hours after the cap has been put in place.

Advantages: The cap is mostly free of medical side-effects, unless someone is allergic to rubber or spermicides. It's about 85–98% reliable. It, too, can give the cervix some protection.

Disadvantages: Some women find the cap hard to put in place properly. Others who have a dislike for touching themselves may feel unnecessarily squeamish about it. The cap has to be fitted by a doctor or family planning nurse, who will show you where it should go, and any change in weight or more than 7 lbs (3 kg) means you may need a different sized cap. Another reservation many women have about this method is messiness with spermicide. If a woman is prone to cystitis then pressure on the bladder from the cap can aggravate the problem, though using one of the smaller cervical caps may be a solution. The cap can interfere with sexual spontaneity, but not as much as the condom, as a woman doesn't have to be at a peak of excitement to put the device in place. A diaphragm or cap can also be put in place any time before sex, as long as more than 24 hours doesn't elapse. If more than three hours pass between insertion and love-making then more spermicide should be used.

The Intra-uterine device (IUD/coil/loop)

How it works: The IUD is a small plastic device which stays in the womb. A wide variety of designs is available, but they all have the same effect. It's thought that it works by preventing a fertilized egg from embedding itself in the wall of the uterus. This means it effectively causes an extremely early miscarriage if there is a fertilized egg — of course fertilization doesn't happen every cycle.

Advantages: The IUD, once inserted by a doctor into the womb, can be left in place for three years upwards, depending on which of the devices is used. It provides permanent contraceptive cover from the moment of insertion, and can be used as a morning-after emergency measure (see p. 132). It's about 96–99% effective.

Disadvantages: These days it's not advisable for young women who have more than one sexual partner, or whose partners have more partners. This is because the more sexual partners someone has the greater the risk of catching an infection which can then be exacerbated by the IUD. The device may cause heavier and more painful periods. If the device is improperly inserted then it can pierce through the womb, or it may slip out.

Spermicides

How they work: The chemical constituents of spermicides kill sperm on contact. They are available in creams, foams and pessaries.

Advantages: Spermicides are most often used to improve the efficiency of another method such as the cap or condom. It's also thought that some spermicides, particularly those containing nonoxynol 9, may kill the AIDS virus, though as yet this has only been shown in laboratory tests. For contraceptive purposes, using them alone may be safe for women nearing the menopause whose fertility levels will have dropped, but otherwise it's not recommended. Spermicides can be bought over the counter in chemists.

Disadvantages: Spermicides can be messy. If pregnancy would be a disaster then it's unwise to use them without other protection.

Contraceptive sponge

How it works: The contraceptive sponge is a small sponge that's been soaked with spermicide. It has to be put up at the cervix prior to love-making, and it has a loop on it for removal. There is some debate about its contraceptive efficiency (estimated at 75–91%), so those very keen to avoid pregnancy may not wish to risk it. For others whose fertility is low due to age, or who wouldn't be bowled over by an accident, this can be a good and convenient method.

Advantages: You don't have to see a doctor to get the sponge, as it's available for sale at chemists. If a woman can easily locate her cervix then this is an easy method to use, but not all women can. There are no side effects, except for the unfortunate few who are allergic to spermicides.

Disadvantages: If you aren't used to locating your cervix then you may not position the sponge correctly, and this lowers its efficiency. Removal can be tricky, as the sponge should sit at the top of the vagina.

Injectables

How they work: Contraceptive injections aren't widely available, but as you may come across them or hear about them you may wish to know something about them. Such injections contain hormones similar to those in the progestogen-only pill. One kind gives cover for a minimum of three months, another for eight weeks.

Advantages: Once administered the injected hormones give contraceptive cover for quite some time, so are useful for those for whom other contraception proves difficult to obtain or remember, or is a nuisance. It's usually only used as a last resort method, however, because the problems tend to outweigh this advantage.

Disadvantages: If a woman develops side-effects from the hormone injection, such as irregular and heavy bleeding, complete lack of periods, or depression, then as it may be months before the hormone clears from her system, there is no easy solution. It can also have a 'hangover effect' preventing pregnancy for up to a year longer than expected.

Natural Family Planning (The Safe Period or Fertility Awareness)

How it works: The idea of natural family planning is to abstain from love-making during the middle of the cycle, when the woman is likely to be most fertile. As the exact time of ovulation varies from woman to woman, and even from cycle to cycle, exact calculations must be done to make this method work. These can be done using temperature readings and charting them, or through teaching by a specialist family planning doctor to read the signs of impending ovulation through examining individual physical factors, such as the woman's vaginal discharge. Effectiveness when using all the indicators of fertility is 85–93%.

Advantages: This is the only method of birth control which is approved by the Roman Catholic Church. There are, of course, no side-effects, and it may help a woman learn more about her own body and feel in touch with its workings.

Disadvantages: Using natural family planning requires discipline, both to chart the cycle accurately enough to make the method effective, and to abstain during the risk period.

Sterilization

How it works: Sterilization is the only permanent method of birth control. It can be performed on men or women; but will generally not be considered until someone has completed their family or is in their 30s. In both sexes the operation blocks passage of the vital parts for reproduction, either ova or sperm, by cutting, tying, sealing the tubes or clipping them.

Advantages: The failure rate for sterilisation is very low indeed (1 in 300 for male sterilization and 1 in 1000 for female sterilization), so there need be no more pressing worry about accidentally conceiving. Vasectomy (male sterilization) is a very simple ten minute operation which can be carried out under local anaesthetic.

Disadvantages: People sometimes change their mind after a sterilization, and although reversal is surgically possible, it is by no means always successful, and the operation should really be considered permanent. There's no physical reason why a sterilization should lower a person's sex drive, and if you are completely certain about your decision then there will be no problem, but there does seem to be a psychological effect for people who regret abandoning their potential for conceiving. Some women get heavier periods after a sterilization.

Morning-after birth control

How it works: If a woman has had unprotected love-making which has involved penetration, and is assessed to have been at a risk period in her cycle, then there are emergency 'morning-after' methods available but she has to move fast. Unless her medical history rules it out, she can be prescribed four high-dose contraceptive pills (two taken 12 hours apart) and if these are taken within 72 hours they are highly effective (98–99%) Another morning-after method entails a doctor inserting a coil within five days of unprotected intercourse (which is virtually 100% effective).

Advantages: As an emergency measure this can save a lot of worry. If the coil is used then it can remain in place for some years, providing long-term contraception.

Disadvantages: People for whom it is medically unwise to take the oral contraceptive will similarly be unable to use morning-after hormonal contraception. Because of the high doses involved, the morning-after pills are not prescribed to be used as a regular method of birth control, purely for emergencies. They sometimes cause nausea, or headaches. The coil isn't suitable for all women either, so for some women there is no 'morning-after' available.

Quick efficiency check

The following figures list contraceptive efficiency. All methods depend on them being used as instructed, because if they're not then, needless to say, their reliability statistics drop and this accounts for the range shown.

Combined Pill	93–99%
Progestogen-only Pill	96–98%
Condom	85–98%
Cap	85–98%
IUD	96–99%
Contraceptive sponge	75–91%
Injectables	virtually 100%
Spermicide	75–96%
Natural family planning	85–93%
Sterilization	virtually 100%
Morning-after Pill	98–99%
Morning-after IUD	virtually 100%

Abortion

Since 1967 abortion has been legal in this country if performed under certain specified conditions, and approved by two doctors. These conditions are:

(a) that pregnancy involves a risk to the mental or physical health of the woman, or any existing children, and that this risk is greater than that involved in ending the pregnancy
(b) that there is a serious risk of mental or physical handicap
(c) that a medical emergency necessitates terminating the pregnancy to save the woman's life or avoid permanent damage to her health. Terminations of pregnancy must be performed in clinics licensed by the Department of Health and Social Security.

Few abortions are done later than 16 weeks and most before 12, when it's a much simpler operation. The earlier a woman discovers she's pregnant, the better, whether she wishes to be pregnant or not. If the pregnancy is unintentional then she, with her partner if she wishes, needs to discuss what to do. Abortion is a complicated issue and often it involves strong emotional or religious reactions. Decisions need care if repercussions are to be avoided. If a woman doesn't feel she's made a definite choice to terminate, and gone over all the questions in her mind, then those doubts may remain even after it's too late. This is why pregnancy counselling is so important. Relief is one common reaction to termination, but that's not always the case, especially for people who have felt pressurized into a decision. Full consideration in making the decision, and accepting responsibility for it, are vital.

Early abortions, with a dilation and curettage (D&C) to empty the womb, can be day-care operations. Later operations, over 14 weeks, involve hormone solutions which induce labour and require a few days stay in hospital or clinic. Abortion is available under the NHS, it's also available through charitable medical services such as the British Pregnancy Advisory Service or the Pregnancy Advisory Service.

Pregnancy tests

There are now quite a few reliable do-it-yourself pregnancy test kits on the market which are available from chemists. Professional tests are available from pregnancy advisory services, many chemists, some women's groups, some family planning clinics and GPs. Early awareness of pregnancy is an advantage for termination or ante-natal care, and with the modern tests results can be pretty accurately assessed within four or five days of a missed period.

Both home and professional pregnancy testing involves using a urine sample, preferably taken early morning, from which the hormone content can be checked. They are simple to do.

Pregnancy

If a woman wishes to become pregnant then she can do her best to be in the peak of health for the event. She and her partner should make sure they have a balanced diet, they need to avoid alcohol, smoking, and drugs for which there is no medical necessity. She should also ensure she is immune to rubella (German measles) — this can be checked with the GP, and if you need a vaccination against it this must be done at least three months before conception.

If there is a worry over possible hereditary illnesses then the GP can arrange for her and her partner to see a genetic counsellor to assess the risks. The man's health is important too if he's to produce healthy sperm, and he too should avoid smoking and keep well to ensure the best chance of having a healthy baby.

Once you are pregnant, professional ante-natal care should begin with the GP. There are also pregnancy and childbirth classes run by hospitals or groups, such as the National Childbirth Trust, which many prospective parents find useful. Pregnancy is itself the subject of many books and childbirth the matter of huge medical controversy which we won't enter here.

Infertility

It's estimated that about one in eight couples who try to conceive prove to have difficulty. Tests can be carried out, but as many people take up to two years to conceive, despite being fertile, it's often advised that people should relax, and enjoy their love-making for a while before subjecting themselves to fertility tests. They may not be necessary, and then merely serve to put intense pressure on a relationship, so allow time.

If tests become necessary, say after 12 months to two years of trying, then sperm tests are fairly simple. Sometimes male infertility can be corrected, but low sperm counts or very sluggish sperm may not respond to treatment. Female infertility has quite a few possible causes, and a whole array of treatment ranging from drugs to stimulate ovulation, to surgery to examine/mend/clear fallopian tubes. It is even possible to remove eggs, mix them with sperm outside the body and then put them back into the womb.

Fertility investigations and treatments can take years and are not to be entered into lightly. There is independent advice on fertility treatments from charitable organisations, such as the National Association of the Childless. They also have support groups for those who want to air their feelings and learn from other people's experience.

Sexually transmitted diseases

Physical contact can pass on diseases. Shaking hands is actually the way most colds are transmitted, and kissing can pass on glandular fever, hepatitis and all sorts of illnesses. Lice and fleas can be passed from person to person. Intimate sexual contact can also pass on specific diseases, some of which can have very serious consequences.

Personal hygiene can't always prevent disease, but it can help. A woman should bathe her genital area daily, using unscented soap or pure water. Any scented product or one containing strong chemicals near this sensitive area can trigger problems, so they should be avoided, and scented tampons should never be used. Using bath oils can present problems for some women, too, and you should never, ever, put disinfectant in the bath water. Men should also wash their genital area daily, being careful to also clean underneath the foreskin where smegma can collect. It's important, too, for both sexes, but especially women, to keep their anal area clean, as infections from the bowel can easily be transmitted to the vagina.

If there's any cause for concern about a possible infection or sexually transmitted disease then immediate help should be sought. Some diseases are fatal, and others need speedy treatment in order to avoid long-term problems, the commonest of which is infertility. The GP may be able to diagnose and help, or alternatively there are genito-urinary clinics attached to most large hospitals. To see these specialists there's no need to have a referral letter from a GP, though it's wise to ring and make an appointment first. Such clinics endeavour to see people as soon as possible.

AIDS

Acquired Immune Deficiency Syndrome (AIDS) is the most worrying sexually transmitted disease for a number of reasons. The virus called HIV, sometimes known as HTLVIII, can take up to three months to show in the blood. Someone who has HIV may not themself develop AIDS, but they can infect other people by having unprotected intercourse with them, who can go on to develop AIDS.

If the immune system starts to break down through having the virus, then it can take four years for symptoms to show. Symptoms include a loss of weight, swollen glands, exhaustion, fever and sweating, diarrhoea, inexplicable bruising and skin blotches caused by a kind of skin cancer. Once the immune system has broken down many otherwise insignificant infections have an opportunity to kill the sufferer. As yet there is no cure for AIDS, or vaccine against it. Treatment can help some symptoms, but there is no way yet of saving the sufferer's life. A woman with HIV who gets pregnant may be advised to have an abortion as the pregnancy may encourage the disease and risk the life of both the baby and the mother.

The only defence against AIDS is avoidance. In sexual contact, semen, vaginal or cervical secretions, or blood from menstruation can definitely transmit the disease. Celibacy or a completely monogamous relationship can rule out AIDS. If such a relationship is impossible then using a condom with spermicide can offer some protection against AIDS and other sexually transmitted diseases, and using your imagination for sex play other than penetration or oral sex could bring different pleasures to the sexual repertoire. If sex toys are used these should not be shared.

A lot of nonsense has been talked about AIDS, and some people have called it a homosexual disease. However, there are no known cases of lesbians with AIDS. If the people moralizing about AIDS acknowledged this fact their own argument would lead them to endorse lesbianism, but they don't, hence it seems their theory is based on prejudice and fear. This is most unhelpful in the fight to prevent such a serious health threat.

It is possible to be tested for HIV. However, as it can take three months after catching the virus for anti-bodies to show in the bloodstream testing may be of little value for someone who changes sexual partners frequently. Those who feel they may have been at risk need to make a careful decision about whether or not to have a test as there can be repercussions other than the threat of AIDS, such as a block to getting life insurance or mortgages etc. In situations where you can't absolutely guarantee your own or your partner's sexual health it's wisest to act as if HIV is present and to take precautions anyway, or you may be playing Russian roulette.

Hepatitis B

Someone who has hepatitis B can, like someone with HIV, pass it on sexually without even knowing they have it. There are three types of hepatitis, A, B and C, and B is the one that can be sexually transmitted or passed on by kissing or contact with another person's body fluids. It is a serious illness causing inflammation of the liver and can sometimes prove to be a killer. The first symptoms are overwhelming tiredness, loss of appetite, perhaps pain in the joints, rather like flu. These come on between one to six months after infection. Then, as with other liver complaints, there's the yellowing eyes, dark brown urine, tenderness around the abdomen and abnormally coloured stools. This phase can last anything from two to eight weeks.

Hospitalization may be necessary during the illness, though in the long run the only treatment for hepatitis B is a healthy diet, with absolutely no alcohol, and bags of rest. It can take months to get back to normal.

Syphilis

At one time syphilis was so common that routine testing was done in hospitals. Now it's comparatively rare, but can still be a serious illness. In the early stages it can be effectively cured, though it's vital that treatment by antibiotics isn't left too late, when it's done permanent damage to the brain, heart and other vital organs.

The initial symptoms appear between one week and three months after contact and the first sign may be a sore on the genitals, the mouth or the anus. This sore may disappear of its own accord, but that doesn't mean the infection has disappeared. Phase two may be signalled by a rash or flu-like symptoms appearing anywhere from two to six weeks after contact. Phase three is too late for an effective cure.

Gonorrhoea

Women may not get instantly recognizable symptoms with gonorrhoea, but if left untreated it can cause sterility or impaired fertility. Some men don't get easily recognizable symptoms either and so can unwittingly infect their partner. Speedy treatment with antibiotics is highly effective, so if there's been any risk at all it's wise to be checked.

When symptoms do appear, between two to ten days after contact, a woman may notice an abnormal vaginal discharge, perhaps accompanied by a burning feeling when passing urine or a pain in the abdomen. Irritation of the anus may also be a sign, as can a sore throat if oral sex was the route of transmission. Men will notice pain on urination and yellowish discharge from the penis, and possibly itching or discharge at the anus. Again, if oral sex was the contact then a sore throat may be a sign.

Herpes

Cold sores are herpes caused by a virus called Simplex 1, and you can get them on your mouth. On the genitals Herpes Simplex 2 can cause similar sores. There is no cure, but treatment can considerably ease the symptoms, and self-help can be effective. Often the first attack of sores is the worst, but the symptoms will return from time to time. When the virus is in an active phase then herpes can easily be passed on.

An attack of herpes is heralded by tingling or itching on the mouth or genitals, perhaps accompanied by flu-like symptoms. Blisters come up on the infected area and can be immensely painful, giving pain or burning when urinating. These symptoms first occur within four or five days of contact. Commonly, as said, the first attack of genital herpes is the worst. Self-help information is available from the Herpes Association.

Warts

Warts are caused by a virus. Genital warts look just like those anywhere else on the body and can appear up to nine months after infection. Treatment is vital. For men warts aren't serious and are easily removed. They usually appear round the head of the penis. For women warts may appear on the external genitalia, or where they can't be seen in the vagina. There seems to be a link between genital warts and the risk of cervical cancer, so prompt treatment and yearly cervical smears afterwards are important. If a woman's partner has genital warts she should also be checked.

Trichomoniasis

Within three weeks of infection a woman with trichomoniasis may notice a thin yellow or white discharge which causes chronic itching and is offensively smelly. She may get no symptoms at all, and men rarely get symptoms of this parasitic infection but tests can show up any problem and treatment can quite easily cure it.

Pubic lice

You don't need to have sex with someone to catch pubic lice, also known as crabs, though that's an easy route for them. Sharing towels, flannels, sheets, clothes, or anything you put next to your body that an infested person has used before you can pass on lice. They live in pubic or under-arm hair and cause severe itching, and they leave behind nits, or eggs, on the body and clothing. Normal washing can't kill off the lice and their nits, but the lotions and shampoos your doctor can prescribe work quickly. Bed linen, towels and clothing should be boiled or dry cleaned to prevent recurrence. However, as the lice cannot survive deprived of human blood, it may be sufficient to not wear infected clothing or use infected bed linen for two weeks.

Non-specific infection

Inflammation of sensitive parts of the anatomy, the bladder, urethra, vagina or rectum, can be caused by sexual infections. Though there are many germs which can be responsible it's thought that the most common is chlamydia. If left untreated this can cause such severe inflammation and disease in a woman's pelvis that she may become sterile. Symptoms common to these non-specific infections are abnormal discharge, pain or burning on urination, soreness and inflammation around the genitals and perhaps a desire to urinate more frequently. It's possible to cure most non-specific infections. Again, women are often symptomless so if there's been risk of infection a check is essential.

Thrush

Only women suffer from thrush, though men can harbour the infection and so pass it on during sex. Thrush, caused by a yeast known as candida albicans, need not be sexually transmitted as it's always present in the body, but sometimes the balance gets thrown. This makes the yeast multiply, which causes unpleasant symptoms such as severe itching and extreme soreness accompanied by a thick whitish vaginal discharge.

Some women are particularly prone to thrush and an attack can be triggered by antibiotics, tiredness, chemicals in or near the vagina or too many hot or oily baths. It has a nasty habit of recurring. Doctors can prescribe effective and quick treatment for women and their partners. It may also be advisable to give medication to ensure that no thrush is left in the bowel.

If thrush is a persistent problem then self-help measures to avoid and treat the problem can help. As thrush is caused by yeast it's possible to neutralize it using another bacteria, such as that found in plain live yoghourt. It can ease the problem to put plain yoghourt into the vagina (on a tampon) several times a day. The acidity of the vagina can be restored by adding some vinegar to bath water, and it's also said that putting a clove of garlic in the vagina can help. Nylon underwear, which encourages a heat build-up, should be avoided, as thrush loves warm, moist conditions. It also loves sugar, so that should be cut from the diet. In itching emergencies a small wipe of olive oil can help calm things down if cool washing doesn't help. Before self-treatment an accurate diagnosis needs to be made, so it is important to see a doctor, but many women know the warning signs from experience. If you use a cap get a new one after you've had thrush or you may re-infect yourself.

Cystitis

Cystitis, like thrush, may be a woman's weak spot in her health and so if she's under the weather cystitis might strike. Pain and burning upon urination, and a desire to pass water very frequently can signal an attack of cystitis. This can be caused by a non-specific infection which leads to inflammation of the bladder. It used to be referred to as 'honeymoon disease', as it can also be provoked by bruising to the bladder caused during love-making. Doctors can prescribe treatment, but as soon as an attack seems on the way a woman should drink a lot of pure water, and avoid coffee, tea and alcohol. Scrupulous personal hygiene, particularly before and after sex, can help avoid this infection, and so can passing water before and after love-making.

Ringworm

This parasite can get under the skin anywhere in the body. It's transmitted by physical contact, so it can also be passed on during sex. Symptoms are a rash which moves outwards or in a circular fashion which is accompanied by severe itching.

Visiting the doctor

There may well come a time when you need to seek the advice and help of an expert. You may experience painful symptoms, or notice some abnormality, and so you may find yourself in the doctor's consulting room, or even in a hospital bed undergoing some treatment.

At times like these many people's assertiveness deserts them, especially if the problem is connected in some way with their sexuality. For one thing we don't have a very good language for communicating about sex, and for another many people (including some doctors!) are embarrassed about the whole subject.

Here are some guidelines to help you decide whether you need to seek medical advice, and what to say if you do.

Symptom check list

It would be wise to consult a doctor if:

- You notice any unusual vaginal discharge, particularly if it's abnormally profuse or has an offensive or pungent smell.
- You experience bleeding between periods, especially if this happens soon after sex.
- You notice any sores, or experience soreness around the genitals.
- You experience pain while peeing.
- You notice blood in urine or faeces.
- You notice any lumps in breasts or testicles.
- You suffer unexplained weight loss.
- You suffer severe itching of the pubic or genital area.

What shall I say when I get there?

If you feel nervous, and know that you will find it difficult to talk easily, then you can prepare yourself by using the 5R formula:

Reflect
Report
Relate
Request
Result

Reflect Clarify your symptoms, and ensure they warrant a visit to the doctor. Few doctors will mind just reassuring their patients, but it's useful to keep a good health encyclopaedia handy, not so that you can read it and become a hypochondriac, but in order to check on any symptoms. Some conditions which worry people are quite normal, for instance some vaginal discharge or some minor discomfort at the start of a period. Also check on whether your lifestyle rather than an illness is producing the symptoms — for instance the menstrual cycle can be disrupted by air travel, stress or anxiety. If your health worries aren't allayed by these checks then visit a doctor.

Report Don't waffle round the subject. Tell the doctor clearly what symptoms you're experiencing, and when they began. If you're embarrassed about approaching the doctor, here are two suggestions which may help. First of all, remember the doctor will have seen many bodies with similar problems and your everyday language will be familiar to him/her. So you should not allow your embarrassment to stand in the way of communication. Another option is to use the medical terminology for parts of your body which can help a consultation seem less intimate. Using the medical words may also help you understand the doctor.

If ever a doctor says something you don't understand then don't think you'll appear stupid if you ask them to explain — if you haven't spent five years at medical school acquiring the language and know-how then there's no reason why you should know exactly what they're talking about.

Relate Explain how the symptoms affect you; what you feel and think as a result of them.

Request Ask the doctor what you want — an examination, some advice, a referral, some treatment.

Result End by describing the result you are hoping for.

It may help to write all this down, and even practice the conversation before you go. Doing this could help give you more confidence, and ensure that at least you don't get lost for words and don't forget any symptoms or questions. For example:

> Angela is experiencing some pain during intercourse, and decides to go to her doctor for advice. Here is the 'script' she prepared:
> I've come to consult you because I find that when I'm making love with my partner, and he puts his penis inside my vagina, it feels very uncomfortable and becomes very sore. The soreness lasts for a day or so. This has been happening for the past month. (*Reporting*). I'm unhappy about this because it means that I don't enjoy intercourse anymore, and find I get really tense, and that makes it even worse. (*Relating*). I'd like to have an examination to see if anything is wrong, or to have some advice about what might be causing this. (*Requesting*). I hope then I'll know what can be done to improve it. (*Result*).

While most doctors are sympathetic and as helpful as they can be, you can find yourself in difficult situations with them, so it might be as well to be prepared for the not-so-good doctor.

The doctor who doesn't listen If the doctor begins writing out a prescription even before you've finished describing the symptoms, you may well feel that you have not been listened to or understood.

If you want to get the doctor's full attention and have him/her know the whole story, then you can use the assertion technique known as the 'Broken Record' and say something like, 'I'm not sure you heard me. . . .' and then repeat what you need to. Check you're not waffling, though — be direct.

The doctor who doesn't take account of your wants Most doctors will listen to and respect any special wishes you have — for instance, you may prefer not to take drugs if there's an alternative natural treatment, or you may want a second opinion. If your doctor discounts your requests without a reasonable explanation that satisfies you, then you can again try an assertion technique. Sometimes the 'Broken Record' is appropriate, sometimes asking questions like, 'I understand you don't agree with my request. Would you be willing to explain what it is that's unacceptable?'

The doctor who moralizes Sometimes, particularly in sexual matters, a doctor feels he or she has a duty to tell you their opinion of your behaviour. If this is not what you have gone to the doctor for, then you could say so, perhaps with something like 'Thank you for telling me what you think. I'd like to know what the best treatment for my condition is.'

It's counter-productive to antagonise the doctor by being aggressive or rude, but it is important that you make it clear that you wish to be listened to and respected as a human being. Similarly, he or she may feel they have the right to tell you their views or experience. Those views may be helpful to you or not, but that's for you to decide.

There's no guarantee that you will succeed with these tactics, and if your doctor seems to refuse to treat you as an individual with basic rights, or you have other reasons to be dissatisfied, you could consider changing your doctor. This is very simple to do. You can either ask to be reassigned by your local Family Practitioner Committee (address in the phone book), or you can yourself ask any other doctor in the area if they would be willing to have you on their list. You do not have to give a reason for wanting to change GPs.

Women have a greater choice than men about health care. Well-woman clinics exist in some areas, and in family planning clinics women (and their partners) will often meet sympathetic doctors and nurses with whom they may feel easily able to discuss things.

Specialist genito-urinary clinics at hospitals are experts on female and male genital problems, and anyone can make an appointment to see these specialists without a referral from their GP.

Health checks

There are regular checks both sexes should make, or have made, on their bodies to ensure all is in good running order. If something is wrong then the regular checks should ensure that any necessary treatment is given early and hence will be more successful.

Cervical smears

Every woman who is sexually active should have cervical smear tests. They are used to discover if there is a possibility that cancer might develop, as treatment at an early, pre-cancerous stage is very effective. One every three years is usually sufficient unless a history of cervical problems, or slightly worrying result, indicate a test should be done more often — perhaps yearly, or even six-monthly. Every woman should keep a record of the date of her last smear, just as she keeps a note of her menstrual cycle.

Taking a smear is a very simple and painless procedure. Using a speculum a doctor or nurse gently expands the vaginal opening so that, using a small spatula, they can reach the cervix and wipe off some of the discharge and a few cells. These are then taken to laboratories for tests. The cervix has little sense of feeling, so unless a woman is extremely anxious about internal examinations, and tenses the muscles, she shouldn't really feel much at all.

If the test result shows all is normal then you can forget about smears for another three years. If the test shows up an abnormality the doctor may suggest you have a colposcopy. This is not an operation and requires no anaesthetic, even though the name sounds daunting. A colposcope is a type of microscope whereby a doctor can closely examine the cervix, take photographs and, if necessary, take a small piece of tissue from the cervix for further tests. So a colposcopy is merely part of the diagnostic process.

If it's felt that abnormal cells on the cervix require attention there are a few options. Laser treatment is being used more and more to remove pre-cancerous cells. If it's felt that enough of the cervix is affected to require surgery then a cone biopsy may be recommended. This involves removing a cone-shaped section from the cervix, and it requires a few days in hospital. Only if cancer has got hold is a hysterectomy necessary. This means removal of the womb, in this case with the cervix and possibly the ovaries. If cervical cancer isn't caught in its early stages then it can lead to death, which is why cervical smears are so important, as treatment early on can eradicate the problem completely.

Breast self-examination

Every woman should examine her breasts once a month, at the end of menstruation. Just before menstruation the breasts may be prone to harmless lumps, so examining at the end of a period is less likely to cause unnecessary worries. It's easiest to do this examination in the bath, as a soapy hand will run over the breast easier. The flat of the hand should be run in circular movements around the breast, moving out from the nipple to the outside of the breast and under the arm. Any lump should be investigated by a doctor.

One of the first tools of diagnosis for breasts is a mammography, which is an x-ray only of the breast. If that shows up a lump then the doctor may recommend a biopsy, which is where some fluid is taken from the lump for analysis. In most cases lumps are benign (not cancerous), but in a small minority further treatment is required to remove the lump, or a larger section of the breast, or in severe cases the whole breast. Early detection of course means that any necessary treatment is likely to be less severe, so a monthly self-examination makes sense.

Testes examination

Men are often left out when it comes to advice about health checks. However, testicular cancer is also one of those complaints which, if caught early, can be easily treated, so men too should watch their bodies. Once a month, preferably after a bath or shower so that the skin is soft, a man should check for any change in shape, size or feel of the testes. He should check each testis using his thumb one side and two fingers the other and then roll the testis backward, forward and sideways. Any lump, change in the skin, soreness or extra sensitivity should be reported to a doctor. As with breast self-examination, if this test is done regularly a person comes to know what's 'normal' for their own body, so more able to judge any changes.

9

Is It Normal?

In any consideration of sexual matters, sooner or later the question 'What's normal?' arises. Everyone has an opinion about this — some people's idea of normality is 'whatever's the same as me'; others consider normal to be 'what most people do'; and yet others take a point between two extremes, to find an average.

Even when you can be fairly objective pinpointing normality is not as simple as it seems. When it comes to defining 'normal' sexual behaviour the problems become very complex. For instance, some heterosexuals assume that anyone who prefers sex with their own gender — i.e. who is homosexual — is abnormal. However, the Kinsey Report, compiled in 1948 on the basis of thousands of interviews carried out in the USA, revealed that only about 50% of people were exclusively heterosexual, 46% had engaged in sex with both sexes, 4% were exclusively homosexual and 37% of men had had homosexual experience to the point of orgasm. In 1948 attitudes were less liberal than they are now — in the UK homosexuality was still illegal — and times have changed. So, if you're looking for an overwhelming majority to measure normality, exclusive heterosexuality isn't it! So defining what's normal may be a useless exercise. It may be more productive and worthwhile to be clear about what is and what is not acceptable.

It would seem fair to say that unacceptable behaviour is anything which exploits the youth, inexperience or weakness of another. And this applies as much in the sexual arena as in other aspects of life. It's unacceptable to put another at risk of psychological or physical harm through setting out to gratify yourself by forcing another to do something against their will. Rape, incest, paedophilia and hard pornography are obvious examples.

Rape

Rape is a crime, and has far more to do with some men's need to express their fear and contempt of women than it has to do with sexual gratification. It's bullying behaviour in the extreme and it is always unacceptable. The word rape means forcing an unwilling victim to have sexual intercourse — though in legal terms the definition of rape is quite narrow, requiring actual penetration.

Sexual offences without penetration invite the charge of indecent assault. Our belief is that any person who ignores another's wishes not to participate is committing an unacceptable act, whether it's actually called rape or not.

We also find unacceptable some of the excuses you hear from some judges or in the media to account for rape — for instance, blaming a woman for dressing in an erotic way, or assuming if she doesn't struggle for her life then she is actually willing. People who dress well and evidently have money in their pockets aren't accused of 'contributory negligence' (i.e. encouragement) in theft and mugging, yet some women have been so accused for wearing 'sexy' clothing. Rape is worse than theft. It is a violation of another human being, to commit such an act degrades humanity. Rape Crisis Centres are available for immediate or long-term assistance to rape victims.

Incest

Incest means sexual intercourse between people who are so closely related to one another that such intimacy is forbidden. Incest laws have existed in nearly all human societies since time immemorial. Laws prohibiting sexual relationships between parents and children, and brothers and sisters, are particularly common.

These law are based on a number of practical considerations. It would be extremely destructive to any family group or society if sons, for instance, as soon as they were strong enough, could oust their ageing fathers and take over their mother. It would be equally problematic if fathers, once their daughters were grown up, could abandon their wives and marry their daughters. There's also evidence that in-breeding can bring out genetic weaknesses in offspring. But other than these conditions, incest is usually, once again, an abuse of power where an adult bribes, or frightens, an unwilling child, who in this case may well have trusted and cared for the perpetrator.

Incest involves acts taking place without fully informed consent which are well-known to be psychologically and often physically harmful. Incest, almost without fail, exploits youth and weakness. Advice to victims, past or current, is available through organizations such as Incest Crisis Line, as well as organizations like the NSPCC.

Paedophilia

Paedophilia is the term used to describe grown-ups having sexual relationships with children, and it is against the law in most countries. Obviously, using our terms of reference for acceptability, since adults are always in a position of power over children, this is an example of the exploitation of power. Pederasts (as they're also known), often defend themselves by saying that the child is, or seems to be, willing, but the inequality of the power relationship between the two makes this a fairly meaningless excuse. One of the jobs which goes with being a grown-up is to protect children, and assist them to become happy and healthy adults, and this should apply whether they are actually your own biological children or not. It's difficult to see how a child's development can be helped by forcing him or her into gratifying one adult's sexual desire through bribery, fear or naïve curiosity.

Pornography

Pornography is the word used to describe any medium which offends our standards of sexual morality — books, films, photographs, postcards, statues or paintings may be termed pornographic. Since different people have different standards, it's difficult to define what is pornographic. For instance, photographs of naked or near-naked women, printed in order to provide some titillation for particular newspaper readers every day, offend many other people. Some people who criticise such photographs because they show a semi-clad provocatively posed woman who's to be viewed only as a body, feel there's a qualitative difference between these and, say, paintings and sculptures of nudes in art galleries. So pornography appears to be defined by more than subject matter. It could be argued that the context defines pornography. A semi-naked woman next to a newspaper story about a vicious rape could be seen as qualitatively different from a study of a nude swimming in a beautiful stream.

It is true that many people get a great deal of pleasure from looking at pictures which show people having sex. Some people find the pictures actually help them to be better sexual partners, and for some, who may or may not have a partner, they provide excitement and arousal. When thought of in this way, it's difficult to find a reason for condemning pictures showing people engaging in what, after all, is perfectly natural behaviour.

So, we will return to our criteria for what is and is not acceptable. Pictures which portray oppression or exploitation of others are unacceptable. This is sometimes called 'hard' pornography. There is strong opinion, although not much concrete evidence, that this kind of pornography has a brutalizing effect on the person who regularly reads or sees it. If someone is so cut off from the world and so lacking in healthy education about sex and relationships that they come to view such pictures as a desirable reality, then it's easy to see how they may stray into unacceptable behaviour. Not only that, but then become confused and angry when such sexual tactics are rejected, and this can lead to rape or sexual violence.

Men are reputed to be more turned on by visual matter than women. Certainly men buy pornography and women rarely do, and in heterosexual couples the issue of 'girlie' magazines may become heated. The man may see no harm in 'just looking', the woman on the other hand may feel that her partner looking at any other female bodies is a criticism of her own — that she's not satisfying or good enough. If it's her own fears and inhibitions about her own body which surface when faced with other naked or semi-clad women whether in print, in TV shows or on a beach, then reassurance from her partner may help remove the problem. We all have to accept, though, that our partners will still continue to find others attractive. It's what they *do* about it, as a matter of choice, which makes the difference.

If a partner's objection to pornography is not a sign of insecurity, but a feeling of disgust at human bodies being portrayed that way then, clearly, an agreement has to be reached between them about how they'll deal with the issue. He might decide to forego that pleasure, she might decide to ignore 'tame' pictures but ban others. It's for the couple to decide where their own level of acceptability lies.

Sexual addictions

Just as emotional problems can show themselves by producing physical problems such as addictions to alcohol or drugs, phobias or obsessions, so they can manifest themselves in our sex lives. If the harm isn't directed at someone or something else, then it may be turned inwards prompting self-destructive behaviour. A nymphomaniac, for example, may be the butt of male locker-room jokes, but an insatiable appetite for sex may well indicate that the person is never satisfied, never happy, forever searching and never finding. Similarly promiscuity may be more of a running-away, or fear of commitment, than just a lust for new sexual partners. Just like the heroin junkie, the promiscuous man or woman needs a regular fix, to be taken high by something else.

Our definition of promiscuity means having sex with anybody, indiscriminately, without respecting the emotional needs of partners. In our society it's not a generally acceptable way of organizing sexual relationships. There are both moral and practical reasons why a promiscuous life is unwise.

Practically, there is more risk of catching a sexually transmitted disease from someone who has intercourse with many people who are strangers or casual affairs. As the AIDS problem increases, promiscuity becomes even more risky. But there are other considerations. The whole purpose of this book is to help people make and maintain relationships which are enriching and fulfilling. Intimate relationships are enhanced by sexual intercourse which can be a wonderful way of expressing closeness and having fun.

The qualities of a good relationship which we have emphasized —for example, sensitivity to and respect for each other's needs — are important elements. Any contact which doesn't include these will do no more than pass the time. We're not talking here about the length of a relationship. We do not believe that the only good relationship is a long one — the intimate and rewarding contact we're talking about can occur in a very short relationship. What is important is the quality of contact. Whether or not you choose to have many partners or one, or whether you choose to have sexual intercourse or not, are decisions entirely up to you. Like any decision you make about your life, you need to take into account any influencing factors. These factors will include your own needs and wants, your own personal history and experience, your own set of values and beliefs.

The desire to find someone with whom one can share one's life in a happy way seems to be deeply ingrained in us. One view of promiscuity is that the person who jumps from one bed to another is avoiding the responsibilities and risks a committed relationship carries, or uses this as a way of rebelling against the morals and values of family, religion or society. If this is right, then it seems a very destructive way to prove that one is autonomous, since it seems rarely, if ever, to lead to a happy and satisfying life.

However, the word promiscuous is often misused by people who condemn anyone who enjoys a sexual life not strictly within the code of one life-long marriage partner. Such people are usually very moral and indignant and will condemn anyone who sleeps with more than one partner, or who has sex before they are married or reach a certain age.

What is interesting to point out is that these people often operate a double standard: for instance they may condemn women as being promiscuous and yet men who engage in the same kind of behaviour are often excused with phrases like 'Well, he has to sow his wild oats while he's young', or 'You can't blame him, she was asking for it'. Women who enjoy sex and who are open about their sexual relationships can be called flighty, or sluts or tarts — men, on the other hand, are congratulated on their masculinity and drive. There is no male equivalent for words like whore, slag or slut. In fact the kinds of words used to describe sexually active men have a congratulatory ring about them — 'stud' is an example.

So before labelling someone as promiscuous, and by so doing discounting and condemning them as bad or worthless, it's necessary to define what you mean by promiscuous. It's also necessary to understand that the person may have some reason for behaving as they do. They may be desperately searching for someone to love, or who will love them, and believe this is the only way of finding that person; they may have developed a life-script which pushes them into this way of avoiding intimacy; they may believe that they have to be this way in order to be accepted by their peer group. Promiscuity may involve some exploitation, but it's more self-abuse than malevolence towards others.

Sado-masochism

Some people get addicted to giving or receiving pain, and search out physically sado-masochistic love-lives. If both partners are willing, and able, to call a halt whenever they wish, then if they find that a mutually satisfying way of behaving why should anyone else interfere? One inherent problem in sado-masochism, of course, is that one likes to be the master, the other the slave, so notions of equality may be difficult to put into practice, and the question of willingness difficult to establish.

Fetishes

It's hard to see how an individual's fetish about, say, clothing could possibly upset anyone else, but yet again, we come back to what other people consider normal. Some may consider those who get turned on by stiletto shoes, rubber, leather, particular underwear and so on, as a bit kinky. It could be said, of course, that fetishes such as these are as harmless as getting aesthetic or stimulating pleasure from looking at the work of a painter. Certainly, according to our criteria of acceptable and unacceptable, fetishes do no harm to anyone at all.

Transvestism

Cross-dressing gets some people very hot under the collar. Not that long ago a woman who wore trousers was frowned upon, and thought to be a bit odd. If a woman wore a man's suit she was certainly perceived to be totally rejecting her femininity. Now, however, a woman in man's clothing is a commonplace sight, even described as sexy and sophisticated. Men in female garb, though, can produce shock-waves even amongst their nearest and dearest. Men still don't enjoy the freedom allowed to women to express different sides of their personality through the clothes they wear, and really that's all cross-dressing is.

Some men find it very hard to express the softer side of their personality, what's considered to be the more feminine side, in their everyday 'male' clothing — it takes a frock to do it. Often men who do get a great feeling of release and sexual excitement from wearing female clothing have had the macho message drummed into them so hard that even though they get overwhelming urges to dress female, their emotions fight with them telling them it's wrong, and that they're somehow warped. Yet such men don't want to *be* women, nor do they generally want homosexual relationships, they just want to let their hair down a bit. Perhaps what this should tell us is that putting men into emotional straight-jackets, making them feel they have to be always tough, always butch, has a backlash.

Transsexuality

The word ascribed to men who cross-dress is transvestite. This is quite different from a transsexual, who will undergo long drug treatment and painful surgery to change his or her body to the opposite gender. You cannot possibly decide to put yourself through such agonies without being in serious pain and conflict with yourself in the first place. Consequently no-one in this country can receive the necessary treatment or surgery required to change sex without first receiving psychiatric help, and a period of orientation in cross-dressing, to see if they can really cope with what they believe they want.

Celibacy

Last, but by no means least, people who don't have a sexual

relationship, who by circumstance or choice are virgins or celibate, may feel they are somehow abnormal. They aren't. Sex is an appetite, but it's not like eating, where if you don't eat you'll die. People can lead perfectly happy and contented lives without a sexual relationship, and such a relationship is only worthwhile anyway if it happens with caring. Point-scoring sex, to bed someone simply because they're available, and to boast to others, degrades both parties. Good loving can make you feel wonderful and wanted. Convenience sex may simply leave a bad taste, and celibacy has to be preferable to that.

Further Reading

Argyle, Michael, *The Psychology of Interpersonal Behaviour* (Penguin 1983)

Berne, Eric, *Games People Play* (Penguin 1970)
What Do You Say After You Say Hello? (Corgi 1975)

Comfort, Alex, *The Joy of Sex* (Quartet 1974)

Devlin, David, *The Book of Love* (New English Library 1975)

Diagram Group, *Man's Body — An Owner's Manual* (Corgi 1977)
Woman's Body — An Owner's Manual (Corgi 1978)

Gibran, Kahlil, *The Prophet* (Heinemann 1926)

Harris, Thomas A., *I'm OK, You're OK* (Pan 1973)

Hughes, Beatrix, and Boothroyd, Rodney, *Fight or Flight?* (Faber and Faber 1985)

James, Muriel, and Jongeward, Dorothy, *Born to Win* (Addison-Wesley 1971)

Lanson, Lucienne, *From Woman To Woman* (Penguin 1983)

Parkes, Colin Murray, *Bereavement* (Penguin 1975)

Pease, Allan, *Body Language* (Sheldon Press 1984)

Phillips, Angela, and Rakusan, Jill, *Our Bodies, Ourselves* (Penguin 1978)

Rogers, Carl, *On Becoming a Person* (Constable 1974)

Skynner, Robin, and Cleese, John, *Families and How to Survive Them* (Methuen 1983)

Smith, Manuel J., *When I Say No, I Feel Guilty* (Bantam Books 1976)

Steiner, Claude, *Scripts People Live* (Grove Press 1974)
The Other Side of Power (Grove Press 1982)

Woollams, Stan, and Brown, Michael, *Total Handbook of Transactional Analysis* (Prentice-Hall 1979)

Useful Addresses

Beaumont Society
BM Box 3084
London WC1N 3XX
Advice about coping with transvestism (will also advise partners)

British Agencies for Adoption and Fostering
11 Southwark Street
London SE1 1RQ
Tel: 01-407 8800
Advice and information on all aspects of adoption and fostering

British Association for Counselling
37a Sheep Street
Rugby
Warwickshire
Tel: 0788 78328
Information about counselling services available

British Pregnancy Advisory Service
Head Office
Austy Manor
Wootton Wawen
Solihull
West Midlands
Tel: 056 423225
A wide range of fertility services, including abortion

Brook Advisory Centres
Head Office
153a East Street
London SE17 2SD
Tel: 01-735 0085
Information, advice and help about contraception for young people

Family Planning Information Service
27–35 Mortimer Street
London W1N 7RJ
Tel: 01-636 7866
Information on all aspects of contraception and sexuality, and a mail order bookshop

Family Planning Clinics may also be listed in the phone book

Friend
33a Seven Sisters Road
London N7 6AX
Tel: 01-359 7371 (7.30pm–10.00pm)
Counselling on homosexual problems

Gay Christian Movement
BM 6914
London WC1N 3XX
Advice and support to gay Christians

Gay Switchboard
Tel: 01-837 7324
Information on all aspects of homosexuality

Herpes Association
39–41 North Road
London N7 6DP
Information and support for herpes problems

Incest Crisis Line
Tel: 01-422 5100 or 01-890 4732
Advice, understanding and support to incest victims or aggressors

Lesbian Line
BM 1514
London WC1N 3XX
Tel: 01-251 6911 (Mon/Fri 2.00pm–10.00pm, Tues/Weds/Thurs 7.00pm–10.00pm)
Information and advice to lesbians

Marriage Guidance Council
Head Office
Herbert Gray College
Little Church Street
Rugby
Warwickshire
Tel: 0788 73241
Information on local services (listed in the phone book), and a mail order book service

National Association for the Childless
Birmingham Settlement
318 Summer Lane
Birmingham B19 3RL
Tel: 021 359 4887
Information and advice on all aspects of infertility

National Childbirth Trust
Head Office
9 Queensborough Terrace
London W2 3TB
Tel: 01-221 3833
Information on childbirth and baby care, and local groups

National Organisation for Counselling of Adoptees and Parents (NORCAP)
3 New High Street
Headington
Oxford OX3 7AJ
Tel: 0865 750554
Information and advice on post-adoption issues

National Society for the Prevention of Cruelty to Children (NSPCC)
Head Office
67 Saffron Hill
London EC1N 8RS
Tel: 01-242 1626
Advice and help on child abuse — where necessary they may intervene, but all calls are treated in confidence

Natural Family Planning Clinic
Birmingham Maternity Hospital
Queen Elizabeth Medical Centre
Edgbaston
Birmingham 15
For details of natural family planning centres

Parents Enquiry
16 Honley Road
London SE6 2HZ
Advice and support for parents with homosexual offspring

Pregnancy Advisory Service
11–13 Charlotte Street
London W1D 1HD
Tel: 01-637 8962
Advice and help on abortion or sterilization

Pre-Menstrual Tension Advisory Service
PO Box 268
Hove
East Sussex BN3 1RW
Information and advice on nutritional aids to overcoming PMT and similar problems

Rape Crisis Centre
PO Box 69
London WC1X 9NJ
Tel: 01-837 1600 (24 hour emergency number)
01-278 3956 (office number)
Information, advice and help with post-rape problems, including immediate and emergency help if necessary. There are other Rape Crisis Centres across the country.

Sexual and Personal Relationship Problems of the Disabled (SPOD)
286 Camden Road
London N7 0BJ
Tel: 01-607 8851
Information and advice on sexuality specifically geared for people with disabilities

Sexually Transmitted Disease Clinics — listed under Venereal Diseases in the phone book

Terrence Higgins Trust
BM AIDS
London WC1N 3XX
Tel: Helpline 01-833 2971
Information and advice on AIDs

TV/TS Group
2–4 French Place
Shoreditch
London E1 6JB
Tel: Helpine 01-729 1466
Information and advice for both transvestites and transsexuals

Womens Health Concern
Ground Floor Flat
17 Earls Terrace
London W8 6LP
Tel: 01-602 6669
Information on all aspects of women's health care

Index